O C L
OXFORD CARDIOLOGY LIBRARY

Catheterization and Interventional Cardiology in Adult Patients

T0177455

► Except where otherwise stated, drug doses and recommendations are for the non-pregnant adult who is not breast-feeding.

O C L
OXFORD CARDIOLOGY LIBRARY

Catheterization and Interventional Cardiology in Adult Patients

Edited by

Petr Widimsky, MD, DrSc, FESC
Professor of Medicine
Cardiocenter, 3rd Faculty of Medicine,
Charles University,
Prague, Czech Republic

Harry Suryapranata, MD, PhD, FESC
Cardiology Department,
Isala Klinieken,
Zwolle, The Netherlands

Alec Vahanian, MD, PhD, FESC
Professor of Medicine,
Cardiology Department,
University Hospital Bichat,
Paris, France

Jozef Mašura, MD, PhD
Associate Professor of Paediatric Medicine,
Childrens University Hospital,
Bratislava, Slovak Republic

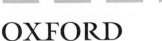

OXFORD
UNIVERSITY PRESS

OXFORD
UNIVERSITY PRESS

Great Clarendon Street, Oxford OX2 6DP

Oxford University Press is a department of the University of Oxford.
It furthers the University's objective of excellence in research, scholarship,
and education by publishing worldwide in

Oxford New York

Auckland Cape Town Dar es Salaam Hong Kong Karachi
Kuala Lumpur Madrid Melbourne Mexico City Nairobi
New Delhi Shanghai Taipei Toronto

With offices in

Argentina Austria Brazil Chile Czech Republic France Greece
Guatemala Hungary Italy Japan Poland Portugal Singapore
South Korea Switzerland Thailand Turkey Ukraine Vietnam

Oxford is a registered trade mark of Oxford University Press
in the UK and in certain other countries

Published in the United States
by Oxford University Press Inc., New York

British Library Cataloguing in Publication Data
Data available

Library of Congress Cataloging in Publication Data
Data available

Typeset by Newgen Imaging Systems (P) Ltd., Chennai, India
Printed in Great Britain
on acid-free paper by
Ashford Colour Press, Gosport, Hampshire

ISBN 978-0-19-955887-2

10 9 8 7 6 5 4 3 2 1

Contents

Preface

Diagnostic cardiac catheterization (especially coronary angiography) is one of the three most important diagnostic methods in clinical cardiology—besides electrocardiography and echocardiography. The world first *diagnostic* cardiac catheterization (in 11 patients) was performed by Dr. Otto Klein in Prague, 1930. This method has subsequently developed into one of the key subspecialties within clinical cardiology—invasive cardiology. This fascinating development enabled the growth of cardiac surgery. Currently, invasive cardiology is a routine part of daily work for practising cardiologists in many countries. In other countries it is rather a real subspecialty, practised only by selected cardiologists, licensed for this work.

Interventional cardiology as a *therapeutic* method for the treatment of coronary artery disease is dated to 1977, when Dr. Andreas Grüntzig in Zurich successfully performed the world's first percutaneous transluminal coronary angioplasty (PTCA). The 30 yrs history of interventional cardiology has two substantially different periods. During the first 15 yrs, PTCA was widely used for the *symptom relief* of patients with *chronic* stable angina pectoris, while during the last 15 yrs percutaneous coronary intervention (PCI—new name used after the introduction of coronary stents) was used predominantly to *save the lives* of patients with *acute* coronary syndromes (especially ST-elevation myocardial infarction). With the newest available evidence from the randomized clinical trials, it became evident that the more acutely ill the patient is, the more she/he benefits from emergent PCI. Chronic stable coronary artery disease thus represents just a symptomatic indication for PCI, while acute myocardial infarction represents a truly prognostic (and—of course—emergent) indication. This shift in minds of modern cardiologists and health-care providers represent a kind of 'revolution' in modern cardiology: the acute coronary care is more and more concentrated in fully equipped and appropriately staffed tertiary centres.

Interventional therapy of the valvular and congenital heart disease represents the third part of this book, focused primarily on the adult patients.

This pocket book is focused on the practical aspects of cardiac catheterization and interventions for the cardiology trainees and other interested professionals (general cardiologists, nurses, technicians, medical students). The text includes indications, periprocedural medications, techniques, interpretation of the results, prevention and treatment of periprocedural complications, and so on. The description of catheter manipulation techniques is mostly short to leave more space for the interpretation of the results in the clinical scenario. The key reading is given in each chapter, but the book is not a scientific but rather a 'cooking' type of publication. The relevant European Society of Cardiology guidelines are quoted in the text.

Contributors

Giuseppe De Luca, MD, PhD
Divisione Clinicizzata di Cardiologia,
"Maggiore della Carità" Hospital
Eastern Piedmont University, Italy

Gregory Ducrocq, MD
Cardiology Department,
University Hospital Bichat,
Paris, France

Elena Franchi, MD
Divisione Clinicizzata di Cardiologia,
"Maggiore della Carità" Hospital,
Eastern Piedmont University, Italy

Dominique Himbert, MD
Cardiology Department,
University Hospital Bichat,
Paris, France

Symbols and abbreviations

↑	increased
↓	decreased
ACS	acute coronary syndrome
AP	anteroposterior
APTT	activated partial thromboplastin time
AR	aortic regurgitation
AS	aortic stenosis
ASA	acetylsalicylic acid
ASD	atrial septal defect
ASO	Amplatzer septal occluder
AV	atrioventricular
BMS	bare metal stents
BSA	body surface area
CABG	coronary artery bypass grafting
CAD	coronary artery disease
CAG	coronary angiography
CCU	coronary care unit
CTO	chronic total occlusions
CVAs	cerebrovascular accidents
DES	drug-eluting stents
ECG	electrocardiogram
ER	emergency room
HIT	heparin-induced thrombocytopenia
HOCM	high-osmolar contrast media
IABP	intra-aortic balloon pump
INR	international normalized ratio
IOCM	isomolar contrast media
IVUS	intravascular ultrasound
LA	left atrial
LAD	left anterior descending
LAO	left anterior oblique
LCX	left circumflex

LIMA	left internal mammary artery
LMCA	left main coronary artery
LMWH	low molecular weight heparin
LOCM	low-osmolar contrast media
LV	left ventricle
LVEF	left ventricular ejection fraction
LVG	left ventriculography
MR	mitral regurgitation
MS	mitral stenosis
OCT	optical coherence tomography
OTW	over-the-wire
PA	pulmonary artery
PAP	pulmonary artery pressure
PAV	percutaneous aortic valvuloplasty
PCI	percutaneous coronary intervention
PCW	pulmonary capillary wedge
PDA	patent ductus arteriosus
PFO	patent foramen ovale
PTCA	percutaneous transluminal coronary angioplasty
QCA	quantitative coronary angiography
RCA	right coronary artery
RIMA	right internal mammary artery
SAP	systemic arterial pressure
STAR	subintimal tracking and reentry
SVG	saphenous vein grafts
TAVI	transcatheter aortic valve implantation
TIAs	transient ischaemic attacks
VC	venae cavae

Chapter 1

History, principles, normal values, techniques

Petr Widimsky

Key points

- World first diagnostic cardiac catheterization: 1930 Dr. O. Klein (Prague, CZ).
- World first percutaneous coronary intervention (PCI): 1977 Dr. A. Grüntzig (Zurich, CH).
- Intracardiac pressures: normal values, arterial/ventricular/atrial pressure curves.
- Haemodynamic variables: pressure gradients, stenotic valve areas, dP/dt, vascular resistances, cardiac output, thermodilution.
- Oxymetry.
- Angiography.

1.1 History

Cardiac catheterization was first used in an animal experiment by Claude Bernard in 1844. The right ventricle (RV) and left ventricle (LV) of a horse were entered via a retrograde approach from the jugular vein and carotid artery. During the subsequent period of experimental catheterization, many important techniques have been developed: pressure manometry, the Fick cardiac output method, and so on.

The first introduction of a catheter to the human heart was performed by Dr. Werner Forsmann in Eberswalde (Germany) in 1929. Dr. Forsmann introduced a catheter to his own heart following a therapeutic idea, that this method would allow intracardiac administration of medications. The world's first diagnostic cardiac catheterization in patients ($n = 11$) was successfully performed by Dr. Otto Klein in the University Hospital Prague (Czechoslovakia) in 1930. It took 26 additional years before this diagnostic method became widely recognized; thanks to Andre Cournand, who was awarded (along with W. Forsmann and C. Richards) the Nobel Prize in 1956. In 1953 S. I. Seldinger introduced the percutaneous puncture approach, which is used with small modifications still today. F. M. Somes developed the technique for selective coronary angiography in 1959. Swan and Ganz developed in 1970 a balloon-tipped flow-guided catheterization technique, allowing right heart catheterization outside the catheterization laboratory (without use of X-ray).

The original (Forsmann's) idea of therapeutic cardiac catheterization was revitalized 48 yrs later, in 1977, by Dr. Andreas Grüntzig—a young German physician (born in Dresden, June 25, 1939), working in the Kantonspital Zürich, Switzerland. He modified the angioplasty balloon first developed by W. Portmann in 1973 for peripheral arteries. Andreas Grüntzig developed the double lumen ('over-the-wire') angioplasty balloon. He tested this balloon in animal experiments and first applied it to a patient with proximal left anterior descending coronary artery stenosis on 16 September 1977.

The two main limitations of 'plain old balloon angioplasty' were restenosis after balloon dilatation (angiographically present in 30% to 50%) and abrupt vessel closure due to major dissection or thrombus (5% to 10%). These limitations were overcome by the development of coronary stents. The first stent in humans was implanted by J. Puel and co-workers. The procedure is now called PCI. Highly flexible, balloon-expandable coronary stents combined with effective and safe anti-thrombotic therapy made possible the true 'invasion' of inter-ventional cardiology to the area, originally considered as contraindi-cation: for the treatment of acute myocardial infarction. After initial attempts with intracoronary thrombolysis, angioplasty was finally proved to be the most effective treatment strategy for ST elevation acute myocardial infarction.

Thus, a 30-yr-old subspecialty, interventional cardiology is one of the key parts of modern cardiology, saving lives of patients with acute myocardial infarction or unstable angina pectoris and improving the quality of life of patients with chronic stable angina pectoris.

1.2 **Principles of haemodynamic measurements, normal values**

The term 'haemodynamics' means measurement and evaluation of some physical properties of the blood (haemo-) motion (-dynamics). Intracardiac pressures and flow are the key haemodynamic parameters. Special formulas based on pressures and flow are used to calculate additional parameters.

Intracardiac pressures are measured usually by a catheter with central lumen introduced into the given cardiac chamber. The proximal end of the catheter is connected to the pressure capsule (strain gauge transducer) with a membrane. The membrane stretching by the pressure-induced catheter tubing fluid column movements causes resistance changes, registered in the form of pressure tracings (changes of pressure during time). System calibration (including the precise positioning of capsule at the level of the heart—usually mid-chest level) is of the key importance to obtain precise measurements. With poor calibration, significant diagnostic mistakes can be made. *Arterial pressure curve* (measured in aorta, pulmonary artery (PA), or any of their branches) has its pinnacle at peak systole and its nadir at end-diastole, the curve never falls to zero value (Figures 1.1 and 1.2).

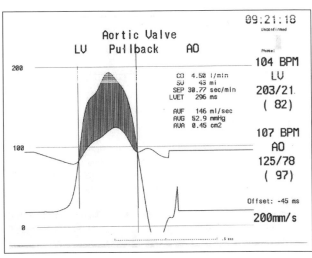

Figure 1.1 Aortic and LV pressures measured during catheter pullback from the LV back to the ascending aorta in aortic stenosis. Pressure curves are computerized (mean values from several beats) and superimposed over each other according to electrocardiogram (ECG) timing. Black shadowing marks the systolic gradient: LV pressure is significantly higher than aortic pressure during entire systole. Heart rate 104/min. LV pressures are 203 (peak systolic)/21 (end-diastolic) mmHg. Aortic pressures are 125 (systolic)/78 (diastolic)/97 (mean) mmHg. Calculated haemodynamic values: cardiac output 4.5 L/min, stroke volume 43 mL, sum of systolic ejection periods 30.77 s/min, LV ejection time 296 ms, aortic orifice flow 146 mL/s, aortic orifice mean gradient 52.9 mmHg, aortic orifice peak-to-peak gradient 78 mmHg, aortic valve area 0.45 cm², body surface area (BSA) 1.8 m², aortic valve area index 0.25 cm²/m², cardiac index 2.5 L/min/m². Kindly provided by Dr. Petr Tousek.

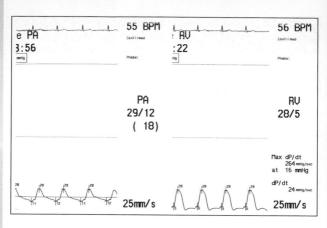

Figure 1.2 Normal pressure curves and values in the PA and RV. The systolic pressures are equal (28 mmHg). Diastolic PA pressure is lowest at end-diastole (11 to 12 mmHg), while diastolic RV pressure is lowest at early diastole (touches zero line) and slightly rises during diastole, reaching its peak (5 to 6 mmHg) during atrial contraction. Kindly provided by Dr. Libor Lisa.

The ventricular pressure curve (LV or RV, Figures 1.1, 1.3, and 1.5) has its peak also during peak systole, but its nadir at the early diastole (when the curve frequently falls to zero pressure or even slightly below zero). The end-diastolic ('filling') ventricular pressure is measured at the end of atrial systole (in patients with atrial fibrillation just prior to the onset of the ventricular systole) and reflects the diastolic function of the ventricle (Figures 1.4 and 1.5). Contractility is reflected by dP/dt+ (maximal velocity of the pressure rise at early systole), while diastolic compliance by dP/dt− (maximal velocity of the pressure fall at early diastole). Their usefulness for clinical cardiology is limited. An atrial pressure curve (left or right atrium, pulmonary veins, or capillaries—Figure 1.5, upper and lower vena cava) has two positive peaks 'a' (atrial systole) and 'v' (ventricular systole) and two negative dips 'x' and 'y' (sometimes also 'z'). The most important atrial pressure value is the mean atrial pressure. The 'a' wave is higher in patients with stenotic a–v valve, decreased ventricular compliance and atrial hypertrophy. The 'v' wave is high in patients with valvular regurgitation (mitral regurgitation results in tall 'v' in pulmonary capillary wedge (PCW) pressure tracing and tricuspid regurgitation has tall 'v' in right atrial pressure tracing). Normal values of the basic haemodynamic parameters are listed in Table 1.1.

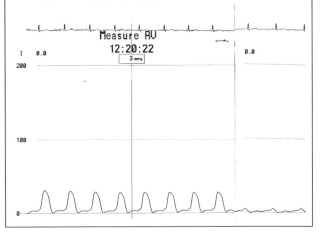

Figure 1.3 Normal pressure curves in the RV (left 2/3 of the curve) and right atrium (right 1/3 of the curve). Note that diastolic RV pressure is equal to the right atrial pressure

Table 1.1 Normal values of haemodynamic parameters

Cavity	Systolic	End-diastolic	Mean
Right atrium (RA)	'v' ≤ 7	'a' ≤ 8	≤6
Right ventricle (RV)	≤30	≤6	NA
Pulmonary artery (PA)	≤30	≤12	≤20
Left atrium (= PCW)	'v' ≤ 15	'a' ≤ 12	≤12
Left ventricle (LV)	≤140	≤12	NA
Aorta	≤140	≤90	NA
Parameter	**Normal values**	**Parameter**	**Normal values**
Cardiac output	4.5 to 6.0 L/min	Cardiac index	2.5 to 4.5 L/min/m²
Oxymetry Hb saturation right heart	<75%	Oxymetry Hb saturation left heart	>95%
$Q_p:Q_s$	1:1		
Pressures are expressed in mmHg (upper limits of normal).			

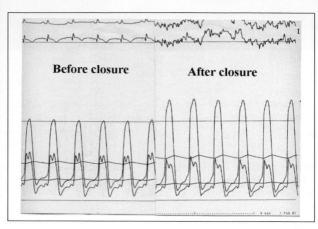

Figure 1.4 Simultaneous pressure recording from the LV (higher curve) and RV (lower curve) in a patient with post-infarction ventricular septal rupture. Left part: before treatment, right part: after ventricular septal defect closure by an Amplatzer occluder. LV pressure increased and RV pressure decreased immediately after defect closure.

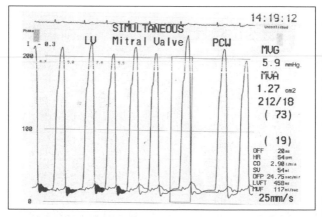

Figure 1.5 Simultaneous measurement of LV pressure and PCW pressure in a patient with mitral stenosis. Due to atrial fibrillation, the 'a' wave is absent on PCW curve, while the 'v' wave is coincident with the end of LV systole. Black colour marks the diastolic gradient (PCW pressure is higher than LV pressure during all duration of diastole). Calculated haemodynamic parameters: heart rate 54/min, cardiac output 2.9 L/min, stroke volume 54 mL, sum of diastolic filling periods 24.75 s/min, LV filling time 458 ms, mitral orifice flow 117 mL/s, mean PCW pressure 19 mmHg, LV pressures 212 (systolic)/18 (end-diastolic) mmHg, mitral orifice mean gradient 5.9 mmHg, mitral orifice area 1.27 cm^2, BSA 1.7 m^2, mitral valve area index 0.75 cm^2/m^2, cardiac index 1.7 L/min/m^2. This is an example how low cardiac output causes low gradient in a significant stenosis. Kindly provided by Dr. Tomas Budesinsky.

1.3 Overview of the catheterization techniques

Coronary angiography: selective radiographic contrast injections to the left and right coronary arteries to visualize their lumen.

Other angiographic techniques: left ventriculography (Figure 1.6), aortography (Figure 1.7), pulmonary angiography, right ventriculography, carotid angiography, renal angiography, and so on.

Intracardiac/intravascular pressure recordings: see Section 1.2.

Oxygen measurements: haemoglobin oxygen saturation measurements (oxymetry run for shunt detection), arterial and mixed venous oxygen content measurement, oxygen consumption and carbon dioxide production measurements (Fick principle).

Thermodilution: cold saline injection for cardiac output determination (Figure 1.8). In the past, dye dilution techniques were used for this purpose (and also for shunt detection), but they are largely abandoned today.

Figure 1.6 Left ventriculography in mitral regurgitation 2+ grade. RAO projection. Kindly provided by Dr. Petr Tousek

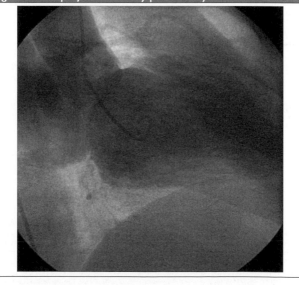

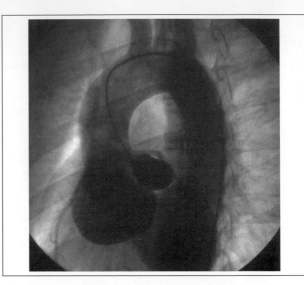

Figure 1.7 Aortography in aortic regurgitation 3+ grade caused by a large aneurysm of the sinus of Valsalva. LAO view. LV is partially superimposed over descending aorta in this view, but thoracic aorta is best visualized (including origins of all three major branches: truncus brachiocephalicus, left common carotid, and left subclavian arteries).

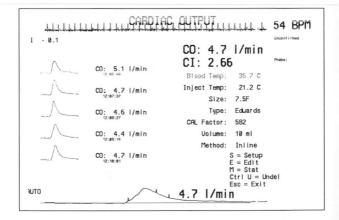

Figure 1.8 Cardiac output measurement by thermodilution technique. Blood temperature 36.7°C, injected saline temperature 21.2°C. Note the variation (up to 0.7 L/min) between single measurements—clearly requiring several measurements to be done and the mean value (4.7 L/min) being the cardiac output. BSA of this patient was 1.767 m^2 and thus cardiac index was 2.66 L/min/m^2.

Intracardiac ECG recording: electrophysiological examinations—are not part of this book.

Intravascular/intracardiac ultrasound: for imaging of the coronary arteries (IVUS) or measurement of coronary flow (intracoronary Doppler), for imaging of the heart cavities, great vessels, and so on.

Other techniques: angioscopy, optical coherence tomography, and so on.

Key reading

Chazov EL, Matveeva LS, Mazaev AV. Intracoronary administration of fibrinolysis in acute myocardial infarction. *Ter Arkh* 1976; **48**: 8–19.

Cournand AF. Nobel lecture, December 11, 1956. In: *Nobel Lectures, Physiology and Medicine 1942–1962.* Elsevier Publishing, Amsterdam, 1964, p. 529.

Forsmann W. Die Sondierung des rechten Herzens. *Klin Wochenschr* 1929; **8**: 2085–7.

Grüntzig A. Transluminal dilation of coronary artery stenosis. *Lancet* 1978; **1**: 263.

Grüntzig A, Senning A, Siegenthaler WE. Nonoperative dilatation of coronary artery stenoses. Percutaneous transluminal coronary angioplasty. *N Engl J Med* 1979; **301**: 61–8.

Klein O. Zur Bestimmung des zerkulatorischen minutens Volumen nach dem Fickschen Prinzip. *Munch Med Wochenschr* 1930; **77**: 1311.

Peterson KL, Nicod P (editors). *Cardiac Catheterization: Methods, Diagnosis and Therapy.* W.B. Saunders Company, Philadelphia, 1997.

Portmann W. Ein neuer Korsett-Ballonkatheter zur transluminalen Rekanalization nach Dotter unter besonderer Berucksichtigung von Obliterationen an den Beckenarterien. *Radiol Diagn* 1973; **14**: 239.

Schömig A, Neumann FJ, Kastrati A, et al., A randomized comparison of antiplatelet and anticoagulant therapy after the placement of coronary-artery stents. *N Engl J Med* 1996; **334**: 1084–9.

Serruys PW, Camm AJ, Lüscher TF (editors). *ESC Textbook of Cardiovascular Medicine*, Blackwell Publishing, Oxford, 2006.

Sigwart U, Puel J, Mirkovitch V. Intravascular stents to prevent occlusion and restenosis after transluminal angioplasty. *N Engl J Med* 1987; **316**: 701–6.

Zijlstra F, de Boer MJ, Hoorntje JCA, Reiffers S, Reiber JHC, Suryapranata H. A comparison of immediate coronary angioplasty with intravenous streptokinase in acute myocardial infarction. *N Engl J Med* 1993; **328**: 680–4.

Chapter 2

Diagnostic catheterization for valvular heart disease

Gregory Ducrocq, Dominique Himbert, Alec Vahanian

Key points

- Echocardiography is most frequently used for the diagnosis of valvular heart disease.
- Cardiac catheterization is indicated to visualize coronary anatomy and/or to answer any discrepancy between the clinical and echocardiographic findings.
- Transvalvular pressure gradient is not precise to estimate the significance of stenosis in low or high cardiac output states.
- Stenosis severity is most precisely assessed by valvular orifice area index.
- Valvular regurgitation is evaluated usually only semi-quantitatively based on angiography.

For most patients diagnosed with valve disease nowadays, severity and prognosis can be evaluated on the basis of patient history, physical examination, and echocardiography. According to the most recent guidelines, cardiac catheterization should be performed only in selected cases where data obtained from echocardiography are inadequate or inconsistent, which is rare. Cardiac catheterization can have several roles in patients with valve disease such as assessment of pressures at rest and on exercise, cardiac output, valve area, pulmonary and systemic valve resistances, measurement of regurgitant volumes, left ventricular function, and performance of angiography. Thus, even if catheterization is seldom performed, it is necessary to summarize the general principles, in particular those which are necessary for percutaneous valve interventions.

2.1 Aortic stenosis (AS)

Catheterization protocol in AS: (1) right heart pressures, (2) cardiac output, (3) left heart pressures, (4) simultaneous registration of left ventricular + aortic root systolic pressures with cardiac output, heart rate, and systolic ejection period, (5) careful manual injection left ventriculography (not with automated pump injector!), and (6) coronary angiography. Simultaneous pressure recording from the left ventricle (LV) and aortic root requires the use of special techniques: either a double-lumen pigtail catheter (e.g. Cook Instruments) or a combination of left Amplatz coronary diagnostic catheter (for aortic root measurement) with 0.014″ coronary pressure wire (RADI, for left ventricular measurement). The use of femoral artery pressure (via sheath) is not precise and should not be used.

The invasive evaluation of the severity of AS requires catheterization of the LV, which could be performed either using the retrograde approach from the femoral, radial, or brachial artery, or using the transseptal approach.

In the retrograde approach, vascular access is performed using the usual technique. Crossing of the aortic valve is an important step, which requires specific training. It is advised to use the left anterior oblique 40° or the anteroposterior view. The preferred catheter is an Amplatz left 1 or Amplatz left 2, according to the size of the aorta. Alternatives are the use of a right Judkins, or a multi-purpose catheter. Straight-tipped guide wires, 0.035 inch, are usually preferred over their J-tipped counterparts. The catheter is advanced until it reaches the edge of the leaflet and then carefully pulled back applying a counter-clockwise rotation while an attempt is made to direct the guide wire towards the valve plane and across the valve by moving it gently backwards and forwards. Attempts should not take longer than 1 or 2 min. When the guide wire has crossed the valve, the catheter is gently pushed over the wire into the left ventricular cavity, trying to avoid a too distal position, which would create extrasystolic beats.

When the LV pressure is obtained, the mean gradient is calculated by averaging the values measured during several cycles (five in patients in sinus rhythm and ten in those with atrial fibrillation). To avoid a pressure recovery phenomenon, the catheter recording the aortic pressure should be immediately adjacent to the valve. Pull-back from LV to the aorta (Figure 1.1) allows for a quick estimate of the trans-valvular gradient measured as the difference between peak LV and peak aortic pressure; however, due to the quality of curves, changes in frequency, and extrasystolic beats, superposition of curves may be difficult and lead to erroneous conclusions in cases of moderate or mild stenosis, when gradient is low, or when using a multiple hole catheter. Finally, the pull-back from the apex to the valve should be performed in order to diagnose the presence of any intra-ventricular gradient.

Retrograde crossing is not without risk, in particular cerebral embolization, and thus heparin (40 units/kg) should be given. A small number of vascular complications have been reported, particularly in patients under anticoagulant treatment, and it should not be performed if the international normalized ratio (INR) is >2.

Transseptal catheterization is seldom used for diagnostic purpose only. This relatively complex technique has had a revival with the introduction of the new percutaneous electrophysiological and valvular interventions. Contraindications are left atrial thrombi, bleeding disorders (including INR > 1.5 or activated partial thromboplastin time (APTT) > 50 s), kyphoscoliosis, complex congenital diseases, obstruction, or agenesis of the vena cava (associated with azygos return). Extreme right and/or left atrial enlargement restricts the performance of the procedure to experienced operators, possibly under echographic guidance. As regards the technique, the most commonly used transseptal needle is the Brockenbrough needle, which is 70-cm long, has a curved tip and tapers distally. A hub arrow on the proximal part indicates the direction of the needle. The catheter used most often is the Mullins sheath, which comprises a dilator and a sheath, and is also 8 Fr. Figures 2.1 to 2.3 show the transseptal technique.

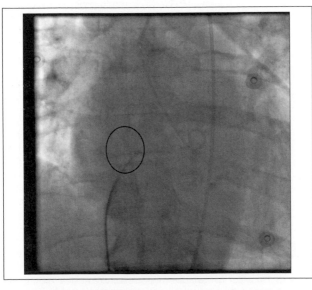

Figure 2.1 Transseptal catheterization–transseptal puncture. Anteroposterior view. The transseptal catheter is at the level of the fossa ovale. The needle is inside the catheter. The pigtail catheter is positioned at the level of the aortic cusps.

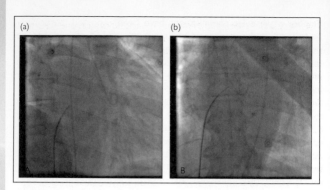

Figure 2.2 Transseptal catheterization–transseptal puncture. (a) Right anterior oblique (RAO) 30° view. The position of the transseptal needle is checked. (b) AP view. When the left atrial (LA) pressure is recorded the transseptal needle and the catheter are advanced into the LA.

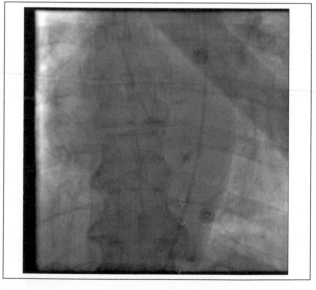

Figure 2.3 Transseptal catheterization–transseptal puncture. AP view. The transseptal needle is withdrawn and the catheter is positioned in the LA

The rare, but feared complication is perforation of the free wall (right atrium, left atrium, or aorta). It mostly occurs when the operator is less experienced, in severe atrial enlargement, or in thoracic deformity. The perforation of the heart may result in mild pericardial effusion without clinical consequences but haemopericardium usually has immediate clinical consequences resulting in tamponade. Its incidence is around 1% but may be as high as 4% in centres with limited experience. It should always be suspected when hypotension occurs during transseptal catheterization. If haemopericardium is suspected, echocardiography should be performed urgently before deterioration occurs. In most cases, haemopericardium due to transseptal catheterization can be managed by pericardiocentesis, especially when it results from only a puncture by the transseptal needle. Rarely, embolism due to a pre-existing atrial thrombus may result in a stroke. ST segment elevation in the inferior leads accompanied by diaphoresis, hypotension, and chest discomfort with normal coronary angiogram has been occasionally observed after transseptal catheterization as is also the case after other intra-cardiac manipulation. They may be neurally mediated as Bezold–Jarish-like reflex and are responsive to atropine.

Assessment of stenosis severity. After catheterization of both the LV (by retrograde or transseptal approach) and the aorta, the calculation of valve area requires simultaneous measurement of transvalvular gradient and cardiac output. Valve area is calculated using the Gorlin formula (Table 2.1). It has several pitfalls particularly in cases of regurgitation, low output, or unstable haemodynamic condition. Despite these limitations, valve area is the most precise invasive parameter of stenosis severity. The symptoms usually occur when aortic valve area falls below 1 cm^2. Correcting the valve area for body surface area (BSA) (valve area index) is more precise: aortic valve area index <0.6 cm^2/m^2 is generally considered to support the indication for surgery. The normal aortic valve area index should be >1.5 cm^2/m^2. Transvalvular gradient is popular, but is not precise; it is largely influenced by cardiac output, left ventricular function, arrhythmias, and so on. In severe AS the gradient exceeds 50 mmHg (sometimes even 100 mmHg), in mild stenosis it is <20 mmHg. Values 20 to 50 mmHg are difficult to interpret without additional informations and especially with these gradients the calculation of valve area index should be a priority. Fluoroscopic evidence of valvular calcifications is an additional sign supporting stenosis severity.

Table 2.1 Calculation of valve area using the Gorlin formula

$$\text{Aortic valve area} = \frac{\text{SV/SEP}}{44.3\sqrt{\Delta P_{mean}}}$$

$$\text{Mitral valve area} = \frac{\text{SV/DFP}}{37.7\sqrt{\Delta P_{mean}}}$$

SV = stroke volume; SEP = systolic ejection period; DFP = diastolic filling period;
ΔP_{mean} = mean pressure gradient.

Indications for aortic valve surgery (ESC guidelines): (1) symptomatic AS, (2) asymptomatic severe AS with left ventricular ejection fraction (LVEF) <50%, (3) asymptomatic moderate–severe AS undergoing other type of cardiac surgery, (4) asymptomatic AS with abnormal exercise stress test, (5) asymptomatic AS with calcified aortic valve and progressive increase of gradient during follow-up, (6) asymptomatic AS with severe LV hypertrophy.

2.2 Mitral stenosis (MS)

Catheterization protocol in MS: (1) right heart pressures, (2) cardiac output, (3) left heart pressures, (4) simultaneous registration of LV + pulmonary capillary wedge (PCW) diastolic pressures with cardiac output, heart rate, and diastolic filling period, (5) simultaneous registration of the mean pressures in the pulmonary artery and PCW with cardiac output measurement (for the calculation of pulmonary vascular resistance), (6) simultaneous registration of the right ventricular and right atrial pressures for the diagnosis of any concomitant tricuspid valve disease, (7) automated pump injection left ventriculography (to diagnose any mitral regurgitation (MR)), (8) coronary angiography.

The invasive estimation of the severity of MS is also based on the valve area index calculation and thus includes simultaneous measurement of pressures allowing for the calculation of transvalvular gradient and simultaneous performance of cardiac output. This can usually be obtained using retrograde catheterization of the LV and simultaneous recording of the pulmonary wedge pressure (Figure 1.5). Although this approach can provide a reasonable approximation of left atrial pressure in many cases, several technical and physiological factors can affect the relationship between the measured wedge pressure and actual left atrial pressure. If an accurate measurement of the transmitral gradient is needed, direct measurement of left atrial pressure can be obtained using the transseptal technique.

The measurement of cardiac output using thermodilution may be wrong in cases of tricuspid regurgitation which is often associated with MS. Mitral valve area can be calculated using the Gorlin formula with the same limitations as in AS (Table 2.1).

It is also important to calculate pulmonary vascular resistances, even if irreversible elevation of pulmonary resistance is more rarely observed currently due to early diagnosis. In addition, the degree of reversibility of pulmonary hypertension is difficult to predict.

As a general principle in MS, as in other valve diseases, complete evaluation is necessary because valve disease is often multifocal. LV angiography is far less sensitive than echography in evaluating associated MR.

Assessment of stenosis severity. Normal mitral valve area index is >2.5 cm^2/m^2, while in severe MS it is <1 cm^2/m^2. Transvalvular pressure gradient is less precise. In severe MS, it usually exceeds 15 to 20 mmHg. High pulmonary vascular resistance (normal values < 130 dyn/s/cm^{-5}) is a marker of advanced MS and carries increased risk for cardiac surgery.

Indications for mitral commissurotomy or surgery in symptomatic MS: (1) valve area <1.5 cm^2 or valve area index <0.9 cm^2/m^2 and favourable characteristics for commissurotomy, (2) valve area <1.5 cm^2 or valve area index <0.9 cm^2/m^2 and high thromboembolic risk (history of embolism, spontaneous contrast, atrial fibrillation), (3) valve area <1.5 cm^2 or valve area index <0.9 cm^2/m^2 and pulmonary hypertension (systemic pulmonary artery pressure > 50 mmHg).

2.3 Aortic regurgitation (AR)

Catheterization protocol in AR: (1) right heart pressures, (2) cardiac output, (3) left heart pressures, (4) aortography, (5) left ventriculography (when LV was not sufficiently opacified by regurgitant aortic flow), and (6) coronary angiography.

Regurgitant orifice area in severe AR is usually >0.5 cm^2/m^2 and regurgitant fraction (percentage of regurgitant volume from overall systolic left ventricular discharge) is >50%. However, cardiac catheterization is rarely necessary and is not more precise than echocardiography in calculation of these parameters. The most important is aortography, which is detailed in Chapter 10. Angiographic grading of regurgitant severity using aortography is shown in Table 2.2.

LV angiography and simultaneous measurement of cardiac output allow for the calculation of regurgitant volumes and fraction, but reliable non-invasive measures supersede the complexity of angiographic haemodynamic measurements.

Aortography can also assess the morphology of the ascending aorta. However it is agreed that non-invasive evaluation, using echocardiography or MRI, provides this information in most cases.

Table 2.2 Angiographic grading of regurgitant severity

Grade	Aortic regurgitation	Mitral regurgitation
1+	Contrast refluxes from the aortic root into the LV but clears on each beat.	Contrast refluxes into the left atrium but clears on each beat.
2+	Contrast refluxes into the LV with a gradually increasing density of contrast in the LV that never equals contrast intensity in the aortic root.	Left atrial contrast density gradually increases but never equals LV density.
3+	Contrast refluxes into the LV with a gradually increasing density such that LV and aortic root density are equal after several beats	The density of contrast in the atrium and ventricle equalize after several beats.
4+	Contrast fills the LV rapidly resulting in an equivalent radiographic density in the LV and aortic roots on the first beat.	The left atrium becomes as dense as the LV on the first beat and the contrast is seen refluxing into the pulmonary veins.

LV = Left ventricle.

Indications for aortic valve surgery (ESC guidelines): (1) symptomatic AR, (2) asymptomatic AR with LV EF <50%, (3) asymptomatic AR in patients undergoing other types of cardiac surgery (e.g. coronary artery bypass grafting (CABG) or thoracic aorta), (4) asymptomatic AR with severe LV dilatation, (5) asymptomatic AR with aortic root dilatation.

2.4 MR

Catheterization protocol in MR: (1) right heart pressures, (2) cardiac output, (3) left heart pressures, (4) left ventriculography, (5) coronary angiography.

MR results in an increase in LA pressure that peaks in the late systolic 'v' wave. The left atrial pressure is transmitted variably to pulmonary wedge tracing, which is the measurement recorded in practice. Although the 'v' wave is often considered the hallmark of MR, this finding is not sensitive for the diagnosis of MR nor is it an absolute value as a reliable predictor of regurgitant severity, because it may be affected by several factors such as the level of systemic pressure, the presence of atrial fibrillation, and so on.

Calculation of the severity of regurgitation by catheterization has the same pitfalls in MR as in AR and is now largely superseded by echocardiography. Angiographic grading of regurgitant severity is shown in Table 2.2.

Very important findings in severe MR are: (a) left ventricular end-diastolic pressure is much lower than the left atrial or PCW pressure ('pseudostenosis' on the mitral level) and (b) systolic (and thus also mean) pulmonary artery pressure (PAP) is increased more than diastolic PAP, resulting in an increased (>10 mmHg) transpulmonary pressure gradient even in the absence of active (pre-capillary) pulmonary hypertension. Thus, in severe MR the evaluation of any potential pulmonary arterial (pre-capillary) hypertension should be based on the comparison of PCW mean and PAP diastolic pressures. Under normal circumstances, these two pressures are equal and PAP diastolic pressure should not exceed PCW mean by more than 5 mmHg.

Indications for surgery in severe chronic organic (non-ischemic) MR (ESC guidelines): (1) symptomatic severe MR with LVEF >30%, (2) symptomatic severe MR with LVEF <30% with high likelihood of durable repair and low co-morbidities, (3) asymptomatic severe MR with LVEF <60%, (4) asymptomatic severe MR with pulmonary hypertension (systolic PAP >50 mmHg), (5) asymptomatic severe MR with atrial fibrillation.

Indications for surgery in ischemic MR (ESC guidelines): (1) severe MR in patients primarily indicated for CABG, (2) moderate MR in patients undergoing CABG if repair is feasible.

2.5 Tricuspid regurgitation and stenosis

The haemodynamic changes in patients with tricuspid regurgitation include elevated right atrial mean pressure and systolic 'v' wave and also decreased cardiac output at rest. The haemodynamic changes depend on the acuteness as well as the severity of valve lesions. Measurement of cardiac output should not use thermodilution in such cases. Right ventricular angiography is rarely helpful diagnostically because of the presence of the catheter across the valve, which induces further regurgitation.

Tricuspid stenosis can be evaluated by the measurement of trans-valvular pressure gradient and calculation of valve area, which would require the use of two catheters and very careful recording of pressure tracing because of low pressures. In addition, the almost constant presence of tricuspid regurgitation can lead to erroneous calculation of cardiac output. Early studies indicate that tricuspid valve area less than 1.5 cm^2 is associated with symptoms.

2.6 Pulmonary stenosis

Typically cardiac catheterization is not needed in patients with pulmonary stenosis, unless the clinical picture and echocardiographic data are discordant.

Cardiac catheterization is only minimally helpful in the diagnosis of pulmonary regurgitation since angiography must be performed with the catheter across the pulmonary valve. However, catheterization is essential for the calculation of pulmonary vascular resistance in patients with pulmonary regurgitation due to pulmonary hypertension.

Key reading

Babaliaros VC, Green JT, Lerakis S, Lloyd M, Block PC. Emerging applications for transseptal left heart catheterization old techniques for new procedures. *J Am Coll Cardiol* 2008; **51**: 2116–22.

Gorlin R, Gorlin SG. Hydraulic formula for calculation of the area of the stenotic mitral valve, other cardiac valves, and central circulatory shunts. *Am Heart J* 1951; **41**: 1–29.

Omran H, Schmidt H, Hackenbroch M et al. Silent and apparent cerebral embolism after retrograde catheterisation of the aortic valve in valvular stenosis: a prospective, randomised study. *Lancet* 2003; **361**: 1241–6.

Sellers RD, Levy MJ, Amplatz K, Lillehei CW. Left retrograde cardioangiography in acquired cardiac disease: technic, indications and interpretations in 700 cases. *Am J Cardiol* 1964; **14**: 437–47.

Vahanian A, Baumgartner H, Bax J et al.; Task Force on the Management of Valvular Hearth Disease of the European Society of Cardiology; ESC Committee for Practice Guidelines. Guidelines on the management of valvular heart disease: The Task Force on the Management of Valvular Heart Disease of the European Society of Cardiology. *Eur Heart J* 2007; **28**: 230–68.

Chapter 3

Diagnostic catheterization for congenital heart disease in adults

Jozef Mašura

> **Key points**
> - Non-invasive imaging replaced cardiac catheterization in most diagnostic indications in congenital heart disease.
> - Cardiac catheterization is occasionally used for the evaluation of pulmonary hypertension or completization of the anatomical information.
> - Oxymetry is used to diagnose and quantify the intracardiac shunts.
> - Angiography may help to localize such shunts.

3.1 Principles of the diagnosis of intracardiac shunts

Left-to-right shunts cause admixture of arterial blood with the venous return to the right heart and thus increase oxygen saturation in the right heart at the site of the shunt and downstream. *Right-to-left shunts* cause admixture of systemic venous blood into the left heart and thus decrease oxygen saturation in the left heart at the site of the shunt and downstream. It is useful to analyse pulmonary arterial and systemic arterial oxygen saturation in all patients undergoing complete (left + right) heart catheterization. Pulmonary artery oxygen saturation >80% and/or systemic arterial oxygen saturation <88% should always result in performing the complete oxymetry run. *Approximate* values for *oxygen saturation* in humans without a shunt are: superior vena cava <72%, inferior vena cava <80% (higher oxygen saturation in the inferior vena cava is caused by high renal blood flow with low desaturation in the kidneys), right atrium, right ventricle and pulmonary artery <75%, pulmonary capillary wedge (PCW), left atrium, left ventricle, aorta and peripheral artery >90%.

Oxygen saturation run (*oxymetry run*) consists of blood specimen taken in duplicate and in rapid sequence (within <10 min) for analysis of an inordinate change in oxygen saturation from multiple catheter tip locations: left pulmonary artery, right pulmonary artery, main pulmonary artery, outflow tract–middle–inflow tract of the right ventricle, high–middle–low right atrium, superior vena cava, inferior vena cava, left atrium, inflow–outflow left ventricle, ascending aorta, descending aorta. The left-to-right shunt is diagnosed when a step-up >6% (difference of means of all samples obtained in each chamber) in oxygen saturation is detected.

Quantification of the shunt. Left-to-right shunt severity is best expressed as pulmonary-to-systemic flow ratio (Qp:Qs). The precise calculation of this ratio requires measurement of the oxygen uptake by the lungs. A simplified method uses just oxymetric saturation values measured in descending aorta (AO), both venae cavae [VC, calculated as $(3SVC + 1IVC)/4$], pulmonary veins or PCW and pulmonary artery (PA) according to the simple formula $Qp:Qs = [(AO - VC):(PCW - PA)]$. Obviously, normal value is 1:1, pathologic values are >1.5:1 and large shunts may reach flow ratios 4:1 to 5:1.

3.2 Atrial septal defect (ASD) in adult

Catheterization protocol in ASD: (1) left and right heart pressures, (2) gentle probing of the catheter passage through the defect from right atrium towards the left atrium, (3) if left atrium was entered, the four pulmonary veins may be gently entered and visualized by small amount of contrast, (4) simultaneous recording of the right and left atrial pressures (pressures are equal in moderate or large defects, left atrial pressure higher in very small defects or when the catheter passed just via foramen ovale patens), (5) oxymetry run to diagnose the left-to-right shunt (step-up >7% between mixed venous blood and right atrium is required for the diagnosis of ASD) and to quantify the Qp:Qs ratio, (6) left atrial angiography in four-chamber (40° left/40° cranial) view, (7) left ventriculography to assess any simultaneous mitral valve regurgitation.

ASD can be first diagnosed any time in the patient's life: from early childhood till advanced age. Smaller defects may cause first symptoms in the advanced age due to the fact, that hypertension or other left heart diseases may increase the left atrial pressures and thus increase the shunt flow. The diagnosis is usually based on clinical and echocardiographic findings and catheterization is rarely needed to make this diagnosis. Basically four different types of this shunt can be diagnosed: *secundum* (at the site of fossa ovalis, most frequent in adults), *sinus venosus* (higher in the septum), *primum* (just above the atrioventricular (AV) valves, extremely rare in adults) and *partial anomalous pulmonary venous connection* (frequently combined with sinus venosus defect). Diagnostic cardiac catheterization is indicated when echocardiography is inconclusive, when a suspicion for an anomalous venous connection exists, when there is a discrepancy between clinical and echocardiographic findings, and when significant pulmonary hypertension is suspected. Placement of an angiographic catheter in right upper pulmonary vein or in left atrium with four-chamber view with X-ray tube positioning 40° left anterior oblique and 40° cranial angulation is the best projection for evaluation of the size and location of ASD or anomalous pulmonary venous return.

Detection of a step-up in oxygen saturation at the right atrial level is not specific for an ASD. Other causes for such oxygen step-up include: ventricular septal defect (VSD) combined with tricuspid regurgitation, coronary arteriovenous fistula draining into the coronary sinus, anomalous venous connection into the right atrium, ruptured sinus of Valsalva aneurysm into the right atrium, and very rare so-called Gerbode-type VSD (communication from the left ventricle via tricuspid orifice directly to the right atrium).

Indications for ASD repair (ESC guidelines): (1) defect diameter > 1 cm, (2) paradoxical embolism. *Contraindications for ASD repair:* (1) pulmonary vascular resistance >8 Um^2, (2) small left-to-right shunt with Qp:Qs < 1.5.

3.3 **VSD in adult**

Catheterization protocol in VSD: (1) left and right heart pressures, (2) simultaneous recording of the left and right ventricular pressures, (3) oxymetry run to diagnose the left-to-right shunt—the step-up >5% between the right atrium (or mixed venous blood when tricuspid regurgitation is present) and right ventricle (or proximal main pulmonary artery in some perimembraneous defects) is required for the diagnosis of VSD and to quantify the Qp:Qs ratio, (4) left ventriculography in four-chamber (45° left/45° cranial) view or in the long axial oblique (65° left/25° cranial) view.

VSD may occur either as perimembraneous (subaortic, subpulmonary, Gerbode-type LV-RA) or muscular (anywhere in the septum, most frequently mid-septal area close to the moderator band). The majority of adult patients with a VSD do not require repair because the particular defect is anatomically small (haemodynamically insignificant) or spontaneously closing. When transthoracic echocardiography is inconclusive and evaluation of left-to-right shunt is necessary, diagnostic cardiac catheterization is required. In such patients, right and left heart pressure measurement with oxygen saturation aids in making the final decision for treatment. The best projection for evaluation of the size and location in most perimembranous VSDs, including those with aneurysmatic formation, is left ventricle angio-cardiography in long axial oblique view with X-ray tube positioning 70° left anterior oblique, and 20° cranial angulation. For subpulmon-ary located defect, the right anterior oblique view is helpful. For mid-muscular and apical defect, four-chamber view is recommended (Figure 3.1).

By this time of life, patients who had VSDs associated with high pulmonary resistance or AV septal defects, especially if operated later, can develop progressive pulmonary vascular obstructive disease. Other possible problems include residual shunts after operation, aortic valve regurgitation, arrhythmias, including complete heart block requiring a pacemaker, pulmonary artery deformity or acquired pulmonary valve stenosis from previously placed pulmonary arterial bands, and residual mitral valve regurgitation in the AV septal defect group.

The diagnostic catheterization and oxygen and NO test is mandatory for any decision and medical or surgery treatment.

Figure 3.1 Four-chamber view for mid-muscular VSD

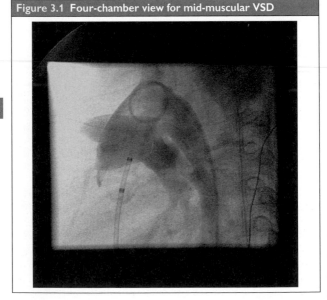

Ventricular septal rupture is a severe complication of acute myocardial infarction. Until recently the only treatment was surgical with poor results and high in-hospital mortality, frequent residual left-to-right shunting and poor long-term outcome. Diagnosis is usually established by the clinical picture and echocardiography. The cardiac catheterization is carried on when an alternative transcatheter treatment is considered.

Indications for VSD repair (ESC guidelines): (1) L-R shunt with LV volume overload, (2) reversible pulmonary hypertension, (3) aortic regurgitation, (4) previous infective endocarditis.

3.4 **Patent ductus arteriosus in adult**

Patent ductus arteriosus can be considered cured by transcatheter treatment or operation, unless rare complications of 'recanalization' have occurred. Some patients may have low-flow shunts due to pulmonary vascular obstructive disease, and this must be established before treatment.

The rare patient who is not diagnosed with a patent ductus arteriosus until adulthood should have cardiac catheterization before being considered for transcatheter closure or operation. When catheterization is considered, the best angiographic projection is lateral view after retrograde placements of angiographic catheter in descending aorta, just below aortic arch (Figure 3.2).

In smaller duct, one could consider hand injection directly to the ductus arteriosus. In very large ductus with pulmonary hypertension, angiography is rather poor. In such circumstances, balloon placement over stiff wire from right heart catheterization is very helpful. The temporary occlusion of the duct for 10 to 15 min as a test with simultaneous measurement of the pressure in pulmonary artery and aorta help to make final decision on operability of patient.

Indications for PDA repair (ESC guidelines): (1) LV dilatation, (2) typical continuous murmur.

3.5 **Adults after previous cardiac surgery in childhood and complex congenital heart diseases without operation**

Tetralogy of Fallot. The successful outcome in tetralogy of Fallot patients who have had defect closure and outflow patching depends on adequate pulmonary artery size and coronary artery anatomy. Patients who have associated pulmonary valve atresia will have had a prosthetic or homograft conduit, with or without a valve placed

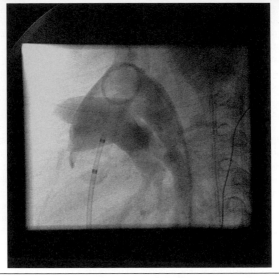

between the right ventricle and the pulmonary artery. These conduits can develop endothelial overgrowth and the valves can stiffen, both causing progressive obstruction to the neo-right ventricular outflow area. These patients should be periodically re-evaluated for development of obstruction that may be treated by balloon dilation or by operative conduit replacement. An additional problem after tetralogy of Fallot operation is long-term pulmonary valve regurgitation.

An anomalous anterior descending coronary artery that originates from the right coronary cusp and crosses the right ventricular outflow may cause a rare perioperative complication. If it is not diagnosed pre- or perioperatively, transection during operation usually leads to death. If the patient survives, left ventricular dysfunction results, leading to long-term heart failure. Emphasis on preoperative recognition of the coronary anatomy in tetralogy of Fallot has lessened this risk, but some young adult patients who were operated some decades ago would have suffered this complication.

D-transposition of the great arteries. A post-operative population of patients who have had atrial switching procedures for D-transposition of the great arteries has emerged over the years. Patients in this group frequently have rhythm problems. Additionally, the long-term effects of the right ventricle working as a systemic pump are unknown. Currently, the arterial switch procedure is the surgical method of first choice for D-transposition patients and the long-term effects of this operation must be assessed. The former pulmonary valve, the neoaortic valve, is not symmetrically formed and dilatation and incompetency of so-called neoaorta frequently develop after surgery. Both conditions require ongoing assessment. The coronary arteries that were reimplanted in the infant may or may not be normal in the future, and serial re-evaluation including coronary angiography is required to determine the function of these vessels. These patients are increasingly recognized as having collateral vessels from the descending aorta to the pulmonary artery. If these create a left-to-right shunt, transcatheter coil embolization will be necessary.

Although the great majority of patients enjoy considerable benefit from surgery, only rarely is 'total correction' of the malformation a reality in the complex congenital heart diseases with or without operation.

Key reading

Allen HD, Franklin WH, Fontana ME. Congenital Heart Disease: Untreated and Operated. In: *Moss and Adams' Heart Disease in Infants, Children, and Adolescents*, Fifth edition. Williams & Wilkins, Baltimore, 1995, pp. 657–64.

Chatterjee K, Cheitlin MP, Karlines J et al. (eds). *Cardiology: An Illustrated Text/Reference*. J.B. Lippincott, Philadelphia, PA, 1991.

Gabriel HM, Heger M, Innerhofer P et al. Long-term outcome of patients with ventricular septal defect considered not to require surgical closure during childhood. *J Am Coll Cardiol* 2002; **39**(6): 1066–71.

Husayni TS. Computed Tomography. In: *Moss and Adams' Heart Disease in Infants, Children, and Adolescents*, Fifth edition. Williams & Wilkins, 1995, p. 190.

Irsik DR, White DR, Robitaille P. Cardiac Magnetic Resonance Imaging. In: *Moss and Adams' Heart Disease in Infants, Children, and Adolescents*, Fifth edition. Williams & Wilkins, Baltimore, 1995, p. 206.

Marx GR, Hicks RW, Allen HD, Goldberg SJ. Noninvasive assessment of hemodynamic responses to exercise in pulmonary regurgitation after operations to correct pulmonary outflow obstruction. *Am J Cardiol* 1988; **61**(8): 595–601.

Nikolaou K, Flohr T, Knez A et al. Advances in cardiac CT imaging: 64-slice scanner. *Int J Cardiovasc Imaging* 2004; **20**(6): 535–40.

Ou P, Celermajer DS, Calcagni G et al. Three-dimensional CT scanning: a new diagnostic modality in congenital heart disease. *Heart* 2007; **93**(8): 908–13.

Podnar T, Masura J. Transcatheter occlusion of residual patent ductus arteriosus after surgical ligation. *Pediatr Cardiol* 1999; **20**(2): 126–30.

Rao PS, Kern MJ. *Catheter Based Devices for the Treatment of Non-coronary Cardiovascular Disease in Adults and Children.* Lippincott Williams & Wilkins, 2003.

Rudolph AM. *Congenital Diseases of the Heart.* Year Book Medical Publishers, Chicago, 1974, p. 49.

Schönenberger E, Schnapauff D, Teige F et al. Patient acceptance of noninvasive and invasive coronary angiography. *PLoS ONE* 2007; **2**(2): e246.

Chapter 4

Diagnostic catheterization for pericardial, myocardial, and pulmonary diseases

Petr Widimsky

Key points

- Constrictive pericarditis: pericardial calcifications and increased diastolic pressures in all chambers with 'dip + plateau' shape of the pressure curve.
- Cardiac tamponade: equalization of diastolic pressures in the pericardium with all cardiac chambers.
- Hypertrophic obstructive cardiomyopathy: intraventricular systolic pressure gradient, small hypercontractile left ventricle (LV).
- Dilated cardiomyopathy: dilated hypokinetic LV + normal coronary arteries + absence of other cardiovascular disease.
- Restrictive cardiomyopathy: 'dip + plateau' pressure shape similar to constrictive pericarditis, but without pericardial calcifications.
- Acute myocarditis: no specific finding. Acute phase—coronary angiography to differentiate it from myocardial infarction.
- Endomyocardial biopsy may occasionally reveal etiology of myocardial involvement in cardiomyopathies or myocarditis. It is most frequently used in cardiac transplant recipients for the early detection of rejection.
- Pulmonary hypertension: present in many cardiac disorders. Measurement of pulmonary artery pressures and pulmonary vascular resistance may be needed to decide about surgery.
- Pulmonary angiography: useful in critically ill patients, brought to cath-lab for suspected myocardial infarction and found to have normal coronary angiogram.

4.1 **Pericardial diseases: constrictive pericarditis, cardiac tamponade**

Constrictive pericarditis. The diagnosis is one of the most difficult in clinical cardiology and this holds true also for the invasive diagnostic approach. When a patient with the clinical suspicion for constrictive pericarditis undergoes cardiac catheterization, the use of diuretics and vasodilators should be avoided and the following procedures should be performed:

- Careful fluoroscopy to visualize any potential pericardial calcifications
- Simultaneous pressure recordings from left + right ventricles as well as pulmonary capillary wedge (PCW) (left atrium) + right atrium to demonstrate diastolic pressures equalization in all four cardiac chambers (this feature is similar to cardiac tamponade)
- Recording must include longer diastolic periods to show the typical 'dip + plateau' (or 'square root') sign (early diastolic marked pressure fall with increase to a high level, where the pressure remains during most of diastole).

The typical right ventricular pressure tracing in constrictive pericarditis showing the 'dip + plateau' shape is in Figure 4.1a and b.

The combination of fluoroscopically visible pericardial calcifications and typical 'dip + plateau' right + left ventricular pressure curve with markedly elevated end-diastolic pressures in both ventricles (exceeding 15 or even 20 mmHg) is diagnostic for pericardial constriction. 'Dip + plateau' shape without proven pericardial pathology may be caused also by restrictive cardiomyopathy (see below) or may be just an artefact.

Cardiac tamponade is usually diagnosed by clinical findings (pulsus paradoxus: abnormally large—over 10% of peak systolic pressure—inspiratory decrease in systemic arterial systolic pressure with little change in diastolic pressure—Figure 4.2) and echocardiography and only rarely is subject to invasive diagnostic approach. When a patient with cardiac tamponade undergoes cardiac catheterization, the typical finding is 'equalization' of all diastolic pressures with intrapericardial pressure (in severe tamponade, these pressures reach 15 to 30 mmHg): left ventricular, PCW, pulmonary artery, right ventricular, and right atrial, all are equal to the intrapericardial pressure. Especially left + right ventricular diastolic pressures are equally elevated. The 'dip + plateau' shape is not present in cardiac tamponade: the left + right ventricular pressures linearly rise during diastole. Cardiac catheterization in patients with tamponade and pre-existing heart disease should be done with three pressure transducers: left heart,

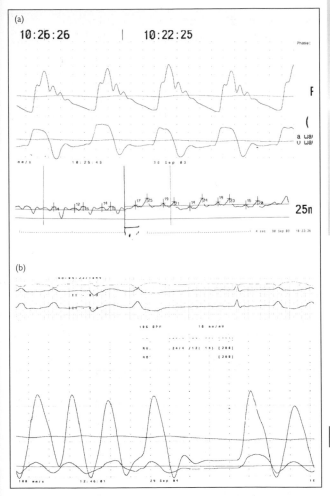

Figure 4.1 (a) Aortic, right ventricular, right atrial, and PCW pressures in constrictive pericarditis. (b) Left ventricular pressure in constrictive pericarditis. Note the importance of post-extrasystolic pause to visualize the 'dip + plateau' shape when tachycardia is present. Both images kindly provided by Dr. Jaroslav Dvorak.

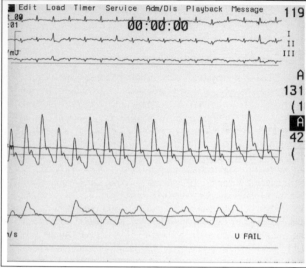

Figure 4.2 Cardiac tamponade: pulsus paradoxus clearly visible on the aortic pressure curve. Right atrial and PCW pressures are equalized

right heart, and intrapericardial pressure. If tamponade develops in a patient with previously normal left and right ventricular function, the use of Swan-Ganz catheter may be sufficient: simultaneous recording shows equalization of the PCW and right atrial pressures. The haemodynamic differential diagnosis between tamponade and constriction can be done based on two signs: inspiratory decrease in right atrial pressure (typical for tamponade, not present in constriction) and dip + plateau diastolic shape of the ventricular pressure curves (typical for constriction/restriction, not present in tamponade).

4.2 **Hypertrophic obstructive cardiomyopathy**

Hypertrophic cardiomyopathy (with or without obstruction) is usually diagnosed readily by a combination of a pathologic electrocardiogram (ECG) and a typical echocardiographic picture. Obstruction is usually dynamic and may vary widely in the same patient—from none to severe left ventricular outflow tract (LVOT) obstruction. The presence and the degree of the obstruction are dependent on preload and/or afterload. The decrease in the left ventricular size (due to decreased preload and/or afterload) or the increase in left ventricular contractility (due to inotropic drugs, stress, exercise, etc.) usually augments the degree of the obstruction. These manoeuvres (e.g. inotropic drugs infusion) may provoke gradient in some patients without hypertrophic cardiomyopathy (e.g. with marked concentric left ventricular hypertrophy due to hypertension), when the measured gradient may be artificially high due to pigtail catheter 'trapping' in the small hypercontractile left ventricle.

Cardiac catheterization is only rarely performed to diagnose this disease, rather it may be recommended in some older patients to exclude simultaneous coronary artery disease. The typical finding in hypertrophic non-obstructive cardiomyopathy may be the 'banana-shape' of a rather small left ventricular cavity with high ejection fraction (usually >80%). The left ventricular cavity is frequently 'obliterated' in the apical part during end-systole (Figure 4.3).

Obstruction in a typical case is localized at the LVOT level and is caused by multiple factors—bulging of the disproportionally large mitral apparatus (for the given left ventricular cavity size) against the severely hypertrophic interventricular septum being the most important of them. Careful sequential pressure measurements with an end-hole (not pigtail!) catheter reveal an intraventricular pressure gradient: systolic pressure in the apical part of the left ventricular cavity is higher than systolic pressure in the LVOT (just below the aortic valve). The systolic pressures in aorta and in the LVOT are equal (Figure 4.4). It is important to avoid a potential error: any fast routine measurement of the pressure in the left ventricular cavity and in aorta (avoiding an extra measurement in the outflow tract) may lead to false diagnosis of aortic stenosis by showing a pressure gradient between the left ventricle and aorta.

4.3 **Dilated cardiomyopathy**

Dilated cardiomyopathy is characterized by the dilatation + diffuse hypokinesis of the LV and normal coronary angiography. Left ventricular end-diastolic pressure is usually increased, causing post-capillary pulmonary hypertension. A mild-to-moderate secondary (annulus dilatation) mitral regurgitation is frequently present. Endomyocardial biopsy may sometimes (rarely) reveal the etiology of myocardial disease. Patients considered for cardiac transplantation should undergo right + left heart catheterization including cardiac output measurements and systemic + pulmonary vascular resistance calculations.

Cardiac catheterization in patients with advanced heart failure has inherent risks: malignant arrhythmias, pulmonary oedema, renal failure, death. The risk can be diminished by minimizing the procedure duration and contrast volume. When the patient is haemodynamically unstable during cardiac catheterization, he/she should never be sent back to his/her room until the haemodynamic situation is stabilized.

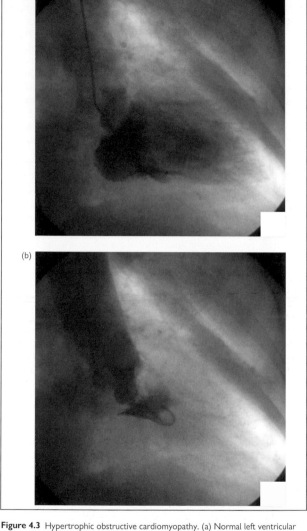

Figure 4.3 Hypertrophic obstructive cardiomyopathy. (a) Normal left ventricular size and shape in end-diastole. (b) Hypercontractile left ventricle with almost no residual cavity at end-systole (ejection fraction was in this patient 89%). The obstruction site between the left ventricular main body and its outflow tract is sharply delineated and clearly visible. Small tubular LVOT cavity and ascending aorta are above this obstruction site. Kindly provided by Dr. Viktor Kocka.

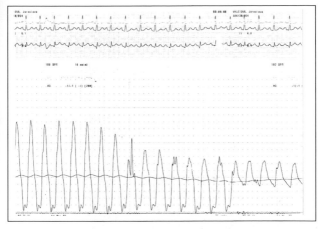

Figure 4.4 Hypertrophic obstructive cardiomyopathy. Intraventricular pressure gradient measured by slow catheter pull back from the left ventricular main body (left) to the LVOT (middle) and aorta (right). Peak systolic pressures are: 255 mmHg (LV main body), 155 mmHg (LVOT), 150 mmHg (aorta). Kindly provided by Dr. Viktor Kocka.

4.4 **Restrictive cardiomyopathy**

Cardiac catheterization reveals usually normal coronary arteries, normal or small left ventricular cavity with mildly depressed or normal ejection fraction, and high left ventricular end-diastolic pressure, frequently with diastolic 'dip + plateau' shape of the pressure curve, same as in constrictive pericarditis. Differential diagnosis against constrictive pericarditis may be difficult—it is facilitated by absence of pericardial calcifications and by higher diastolic pressures in the left compared to the right ventricle. Myocardial biopsy may sometimes help to elucidate the underlying cause (e.g. amyloid disease, fibrosis, etc.).

4.5 **Acute myocarditis**

Acute myocarditis has no specific picture during cardiac catheterization. However, invasive examination may frequently contribute to this diagnosis indirectly by excluding other causes of acute heart failure (e.g. myocardial infarction). Acute myocarditis can have any of the following findings during cardiac catheterization: diffuse left ventricular hypokinesis (as in dilated cardiomyopathy), regional akinesis (as in myocardial infarction, however, the location does not reflect the perfusion bed of any coronary artery), or no visible abnormality (in mild cases). Coronary arteries are normal.

Endomyocardial biopsy may contribute to the diagnosis of acute myocarditis. However, in many patients, this is not the case. If endomyocardial biopsy is indicated, it should always be performed in a centre with large experience in this procedure (e.g. a centre performing heart transplant procedures)—this is especially important for the interpretation of the histology (should always be interpreted by a pathologist with large experience in myocardial biopsies).

4.6 **Stress-induced myocardial stunning (apical ballooning, Tako-Tsubo)**

Acute onset of left ventricular apical akinesis or dyskinesis (mimicking acute myocardial infarction—Figure 4.5) with hyperkinesis of basal segments and normal coronary angiogram and with subsequent normalization of the left ventricular wall motion during cca 1 week is diagnostic for this poorly defined entity.

4.7 **Pulmonary hypertension: cor pulmonale**

Pulmonary hypertension is defined as the pulmonary arterial pressure increase above 30/12/20 mmHg (systolic/diastolic/mean pressure). The cause can be either (a) passive distally to the pulmonary capillaries—so-called *post-capillary pulmonary hypertension* (increased pressure in the left atrium is passively transferred to the pulmonary veins and capillaries—for example, in left ventricular failure or mitral valve

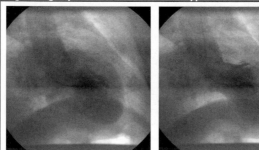

Figure 4.5 Stress-induced myocardial stunning (apical ballooning, Tako-Tsubo). Left: Normal diastolic LV shape. Right: large apical akinesis with basal hyperkinesis

disease) or (b) active proximally to the pulmonary capillaries, usually on the level of pulmonary arterioles—so-called *pre-capillary pulmonary hypertension* (generalized pulmonary vasoconstriction—usually of hypoxic origin)—Figure 4.6. Both types can be combined—so-called *mixed pulmonary hypertension* (Table 4.1). Pressure values in mild pulmonary hypertension are usually below 45/20/30 mmHg, in severe pulmonary hypertension (over 70/40/50 mmHg) may sometimes reach the systemic levels (systolic pulmonary artery pressure up to 120 mmHg).

Three examples with the same values of pulmonary artery pressures and different values of the PCW pressures are given for the better understanding:

- Pre-capillary hypertension: pulmonary artery (systolic/diastolic/mean) 60/30/42 mmHg, mean PCW pressure 8 mmHg.
- Post-capillary hypertension: pulmonary artery (systolic/diastolic/mean) 60/30/42 mmHg, mean PCW pressure 27 mmHg.
- Mixed hypertension: pulmonary artery (systolic/diastolic/mean) 60/30/42 mmHg, mean PCW pressure 18 mmHg.

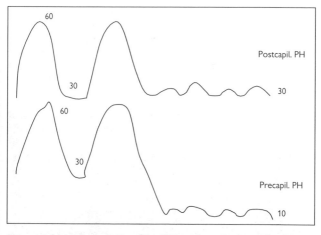

Figure 4.6 Schematic visualization of the difference between post-capillary (upper curve) and pre-capillary (lower curve) pulmonary hypertension. Left: Swan-Ganz catheter balloon deflated–pulmonary artery systolic/diastolic pressure curve displayed. Right: Swan-Ganz catheter balloon inflated–pulmonary capillary wedge pressure curve displayed.

Table 4.1 Definition (differential diagnosis) of the pre-capillary, post-capillary, and mixed pulmonary hypertension

	Diastolic pulmonary artery pressure (PAd)	Mean PCW pressure	Difference PAd – PCW
Pre-capillary	>12	≤12	>5
Post-capillary	>12	>12	<5
Mixed	>12	>12	>5

Some authors use so-called *transpulmonary pressure gradient* (instead of the difference PAd – PCW): calculated as the difference PAm – PCW (mean pulmonary arterial pressure minus mean PCW pressure). Critical value (the last column in Table 4.1) in this case is not 5 mmHg, but 10 mmHg. Otherwise the table can be used similarly.

Pulmonary arterial pressure is usually measured by the *balloon-tipped flow-directed (Swan-Ganz) catheter*. This catheter has usually triple lumen + thermistor on the tip. One lumen has distal end at the catheter tip (and serves thus for the pressure measurements distal to the balloon—typically in the pulmonary artery), second lumen has distal end on the catheter side 20 cm proximally from the tip (i.e. usually in the right atrium), and the third lumen serves for the balloon inflation. Thermistor measures the blood temperature change during the passage of saline bolus through the right heart—*thermodilution method for the measurement of cardiac output*—Figure 1.8. Swan-Ganz catheter may be introduced via any vein (most frequently v. jugularis) to the right atrium. The balloon on the tip is inflated with 1 to 1.5 mL of air and the catheter is slowly advanced: the inflated balloon 'floats' with blood stream through the right heart to the pulmonary artery branch of the same diameter as the balloon diameter—usually one of the (sub)segmental branches. Here the balloon occludes this branch and via its distal central lumen can measure the pressure distal to the balloon-obstructed pulmonary artery branch. This pressure is equal to the pulmonary capillary pressure, left atrial pressure and in the absence of mitral valve disease also equal to the left ventricular filling pressure. The pressure measured this way is called 'PCW pressure' and is largely used to substitute direct left atrial pressure measurement (which requires transseptal approach).

Pulmonary floating catheter should be used by experienced personnel—otherwise it could cause serious *complications*: pulmonary haemorrhage (frequently fatal, caused by inadvertent balloon inflation at too distal pulmonary artery branch with smaller diameter than the balloon resulting in pulmonary artery rupture to the pulmonary parenchyma) or pulmonary infarction (by leaving balloon inflated for too long in a segmental branch). Other complications may include ventricular arrhythmias (during right ventricular passage), tricuspid valve damage (by inadvertent retrieval of the catheter with balloon inflated instead of deflated). Most frequent problem is misinterpretation (e.g. poor system calibration) or no interpretation (and thus the catheter was used unnecessarily) of the results.

Cor pulmonale is the term, classically used by pathologists or old clinicians for the situation, when right ventricular hypertrophy is caused by pre-capillary pulmonary hypertension resulting from severe chronic hypoxemia in advanced stages of pulmonary diseases. Right heart catheterization is the most precise way to establish this diagnosis including its severity and potential reversibility. Pulmonary hypertension in true cor pulmonale (e.g. in patients with chronic obstructive pulmonary disease or pulmonary interstitial fibrosis) is almost never severe, it is mostly mild to moderate hypertension. Cor pulmonale is much less frequent today when compared with 20 to 30 yrs ago. Some authors label thromboembolic pulmonary hypertension also as cor pulmonale, but we believe this should be a distinct entity (see Section 4.8).

4.8 **Pulmonary embolism**

Pulmonary angiography was for many years the golden standard for the diagnosis of acute pulmonary embolism. Nowadays, modern CT scanners offer similar diagnostic accuracy non-invasively, and pulmonary angiography is less frequently used for this purpose. However, we use pulmonary angiography quite frequently in situations where a patient is presented by emergency ambulance directly to the catheterization laboratory (usually with working diagnosis of acute myocardial infarction), and we have clinical suspicion for acute pulmonary embolism (either after coronary angiography showed normal finding or sometimes even before coronary angiography is started). In these emergent situations, pulmonary angiography (done selectively by two separate contrast injections: to the right and to the left pulmonary artery) is a quick and safe method, leading immediately to the diagnosis. Fresh pulmonary emboli are visualized as multiple, gross, sharply delineated, frequently irregular filling defects in the pulmonary arterial tree—Figure 4.7.

Pulmonary arterial pressure during the first episode of acute pulmonary embolism never exceeds 50 mmHg (systolic) or 35 mmHg (diastolic) values. Higher pressure measured during acute pulmonary embolism is a sign of pre-existing chronic pulmonary hypertension. Right ventricular end-diastolic and right atrial mean pressures are usually markedly increased in massive pulmonary embolism.

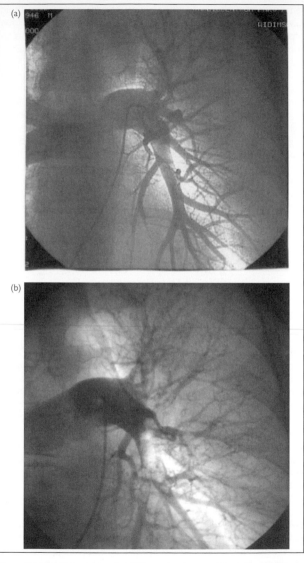

Figure 4.7 Pulmonary angiography. (a) Normal angiogram of the main pulmonary artery and the left pulmonary artery tree. (b) Large acute pulmonary embolus occluding the left lower lobe + lingular branches.

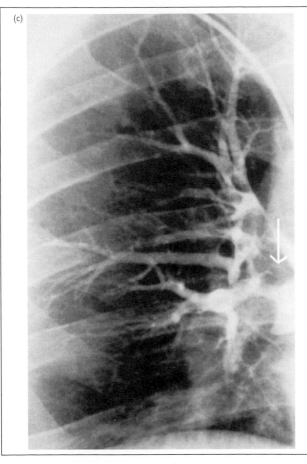

Figure 4.7 *(contd)* (c) Acute pulmonary embolus in two large fragments subtotally occluding the right upper lobe branch and right lower lobe branch.

Chronic thromboembolic pulmonary hypertension may be very severe; the pulmonary pressures sometimes reach the systemic values. Pulmonary angiography may be helpful in differential diagnosis against other possible causes of severe pulmonary hypertension. As with all patients with severe pulmonary hypertension, pulmonary angiography should be done very cautiously: first contrast injection should be done manually with only 15 to 20 mL of contrast. This is safe and in patients with low cardiac output allows sufficient opacification (thus, pump injection of larger contrast volume can be avoided). Only when the hand injection does not result in good quality image (i.e. in patients with normal cardiac output), pump injection of 30 to 40 mL of contrast (15 to 20 mL/s) selectively to the right and later to the left (or vice versa) pulmonary artery can be used.

Right heart catheterization in acute pulmonary embolism should be performed via jugular or subclavian vein to avoid the risk of femoral–iliac–inferior vena cava thrombus dislodgement during catheter passage. We prefer to use ventriculographic pigtail catheter 5 to 6 F, others use special side hole angiographic catheters (NIH or Berman) or Swan-Ganz angiographic catheter. The catheter tip should be positioned near the origin of the lower lobe vessels. Description of the pulmonary angiogram should always include all segmental branches. Right upper lobe apical, posterior, and anterior segmental branches are well visualized from anteroposterior view. Right middle lobe branch is superimposed over right lower lobe branch and thus lateral view is needed to visualize the right middle lobe branch. Right lower lobe branches—anterobasal, mediobasal, laterobasal, and posterobasal (biggest one)—are well seen from anteroposterior view. Only superior segmental branch in the right lower lobe area needs lateral view for optimal visualization. Left lower lobe branches—anteromedial, laterobasal, posterobasal, and superior—partially overlap in the anteroposterior (AP) view and lateral view separates them clearly. AP view is sufficient for the remaining segmental branches of the left pulmonary artery: two lingular (superior and inferior), and three to left upper lobe (anterior, apical, and posterior).

Table 4.2 summarizes the differential diagnostic features of acute vs. chronic pulmonary embolism vs. primary pulmonary hypertension.

4.9 **Primary pulmonary hypertension**

Right heart catheterization and pulmonary angiography is usually used to confirm the diagnosis after the suspicion was expressed by non-invasive tests. When patient is sent for cardiac catheterization with this diagnosis, the procedure should be done in a centre with this specific experience and may be combined with pharmacologic testing of pulmonary pressure reactivity. Pre-capillary pulmonary hypertension is usually severe and pulmonary angiography shows near–normal finding (experienced angiographer can describe peripheral vascular pruning and absence of pulmonary capillary blush).

Table 4.2 Angiographic and haemodynamic findings in pulmonary embolism and primary pulmonary hypertension

	Acute pulmonary embolism (first episode)	Chronic thrombo-embolic pulmonary hypertension	Primary pulmonary hypertension
Pulmonary angiography	Multiple sharply delineated distinct filling defects	Enlargement of central pulmonary arteries, 'pouching' abnormalities (branches ostial amputations) or band-like constrictions (critical stenoses), gross intimal irregularities. These findings are bilateral, but not symmetric.	Normal (or dilated) central pulmonary arteries and global pruning of the small arteries, absence of normal arteriolar-capillary blush. All these findings are bilateral and symmetric.
Haemodynamic findings	PAs 30 to 49 mmHg PCW < 12 mmHg PAd – PCW > 5 mmHg	PAs > 50 mmHg PCW < 12 mmHg PAd – PCW > 10 mmHg	PAs > 50 mmHg PCW < 12 mmHg PAd – PCW > 10 mmHg

Key reading

American College of Cardiology/European Society of Cardiology Clinical Expert Consensus Document on Hypertrophic Cardiomyopathy. *Eur Heart J* 2003; **24**: 1965–91.

Auger W, Moser K, Peterson KL. Catheterization and angiography in pulmonary hypertension. In: *Cardiac Catheterization*, edited by Peterson KL, Nicod P. W.B. Saunders Company, Philadelphia, 1997, pp. 401–14.

Baim D (editor). *Grossman's Cardiac Catheterization, Angiography and Intervention*, Seventh edition. Lippincott Williams & Wilkins, Philadelphia, 2006.

Guidelines on diagnosis and management of acute pulmonary embolism. Task Force of the European Society of Cardiology. *Eur Heart J* 2000; **21**: 1301–36.

Guidelines on diagnosis and treatment of pulmonary arterial hypertension. Task Force of the European Society of Cardiology. *Eur Heart J* 2004; **25**: 2243–78.

Guidelines on the diagnosis and management of the pericardial diseases. Task Force of the European Society of Cardiology. *Eur Heart J* 2004; **25**: 587–610.

Polikar R, Nicod P, Shabetai R. Catheterization and angiography in restrictive and constrictive disorders of the heart. In: *Cardiac Catheterization*, edited by Peterson KL, Nicod P. W.B. Saunders Company, Philadelphia, 1997, pp. 376–400.

Shabetai R, Bhargava V, Nicod P. Cardiac catheterization and angiography in dilated cardiomyopathy and heart failure. In: *Cardiac Catheterization*, edited by Peterson KL, Nicod P. W.B. Saunders Company, Philadelphia, 1997, pp. 352–63.

Chapter 5

Coronary angiography and other intracoronary diagnostic techniques

Petr Widimsky

Key points

- Coronary angiography (CAG) with PCI is urgently indicated to improve the prognosis in most patients with acute coronary syndromes.
- CAG is electively indicated in chronic stable angina patients willing to have symptom relief.
- CAG is only rarely indicated in asymptomatic stable patients.

5.1 Indications and contraindications for CAG

CAG in experienced hands is a safe procedure even when done in severely ill patients with acute myocardial infarction. On the other hand, an inexperienced low volume operator may be more prone to complications. Thus, the indications for CAG in high volume centres are wide and the indication threshold low—especially in patients admitted for acute chest pain, dyspnoea, shock, or other acute condition. In these acute situations, early CAG with subsequent percutaneous coronary interventions (PCI) is frequently the life-saving procedure. Situation is different in chronic stable patients, in whom PCI is known to relieve their symptoms, but does not change their generally good prognosis. Thus, chronic stable patients should undergo CAG mainly when they have significant symptoms.

Indications for emergent CAG (i.e. immediate, no later than 2 h after presentation:

- ST elevations ≥ 2 mm in at least two contiguous electrocardiogram (ECG) leads with symptoms suggestive of acute myocardial infarction
- New onset bifascicular block (LBBB or RBBB + LAH or RBBB + LPH) with symptoms suggestive of acute myocardial infarction

- ST depressions ≥ 2 mm in at least two contiguous ECG leads with symptoms suggestive of acute myocardial infarction
- Cardiogenic shock or progressive haemodynamic deterioration with clinical suspicion for acute myocardial infarction (irrespective of ECG)
- Recurrence of ischemia despite optimal medical therapy in any other form of acute coronary syndrome.

Indications for early CAG (within several days):

- Other forms of acute coronary syndromes with documented high-to-intermediate risk stabilized on initial medical therapy
- Stable angina pectoris CCS class IV.

Indications for elective CAG:

- Unstable angina with low-risk characteristics (negative troponin, normal or non-specific ECG, no diabetes)
- Stable angina pectoris CCS class II–III
- Differential diagnostic need when the result of CAG will influence the treatment.

Questionable indication for elective CAG:

- Documented stress-induced ischemia in a stable asymptomatic patient.

Contraindications for CAG:

There is no contraindication for CAG in ongoing acute myocardial infarction. In elective setting (including stabilized unstable angina), few relative contraindications exist:

- Renal failure
- Known allergy to currently available contrast media (history of allergy to ancient contrast media used >20 yrs ago usually does not represent a real problem for modern contrast media use)
- Multiple myeloma
- Lack of patient cooperation.

5.2 Pre-catheterization evaluation of the patient, periprocedural medication, contrast agents

The patient should understand the benefits and risks of the procedure. Thus, a detailed *interview* between the patient and the physician is essential. *Written informed consent* is legally requested in most countries.

ECG is usually the only examination before emergent CAG in evolving myocardial infarction. More examinations are usually done *before elective CAG*: laboratory testing (creatinin, blood counts, glucose, cholesterol, natrium, potassium, urine analysis etc.), stress testing, chest X- ray, echocardiography.

Periprocedural medication. Patients with *acute coronary syndromes* receive multiple drugs for this diagnosis—especially full anti-thrombotic medication (aspirin, heparin, clopidogrel, etc.). Anticoagulation therapy (heparin) in high risk acute coronary syndrome must continue until the time of CAG and during the procedure. Discontinuation of heparin before CAG may result in rebound hypercoagulation leading to periprocedural myocardial infarction. *Chronic stable patients* undergoing elective CAG use aspirin. Most cath-labs use small bolus dose of heparin (40 units per kg body weight) at the beginning of elective CAG procedure to prevent catheter clotting (which may lead to disastrous complications—especially stroke). We sometimes avoid heparin in low-weighted females (who are at highest risk of bleeding complications) when we expect a very short procedure from the femoral approach. Heparin should be always used with radial approach. Clopidogrel is used in many cath-labs as a routine pre-treatment before elective CAG and is recommended by the ESC guidelines. However, the PRAGUE-8 trial demonstrated that clopidogrel may be safely used after CAG only selectively to those patients, who undergo ad-hoc PCI.

The *contrast agents* used. *High-osmolar ionic* contrast agents used in the past (ratio-1.5 ionic compounds, e.g. Renografin®, Conray®) caused sometimes severe allergic reactions including anaphylactic shock and death. This almost disappeared in the last 15 yrs with the use of modern contrast agents. *Ratio-3 lower-osmolarity ionic* contrast materials (e.g. ioxaglate—Hexabrix®, Telebrix®) have osmolarity cca twice that of blood and thus have much lower incidence of side effects. The newest *non-ionic, ratio-3, low-osmolar* contrast agents (e.g. iopamidol—Isovue®, iohexol—Omnipaque®, ioversol—Optiray®, etc.) have some physiologic (functional) advantages: they do not alter ventricular function and coronary flow, and they do influence the renal function to a lesser extent. This seems to be even better for the latest *ratio-6 non-ionic dimeric* compound iodixanol (Visipaque®).

However, the non-ionic agents failed to improve the hard clinical end points in the randomized trials, when compared to ionic contrast agents with lower osmolarity. The choice of a specific low-osmolar contrast agent (ionic vs. non-ionic, different manufacturers) is thus less important today. The contrast volume used influences possible complications (especially in patients with depressed renal function). CAG can be done with the use of 50 to 100 mL of contrast and even when left ventriculography is added, the total contrast volume is almost always below 120 mL. These volumes only rarely cause clini-cal complications. Contrast selection may be more important in the PCI setting, when in a long complex procedure volumes up to 400 to

500 mL may occasionally be needed. With these volumes, the risk of complications (especially renal failure) is already substantial and the use of low-osmolar, non-ionic contrast may be advisable especially for patients with diabetes or with pre-existing renal insufficiency and for acute myocardial infarction patients.

5.3 Access site, material, techniques, post-catheterization care

Arterial access. The access site is first anesthetized by subcutaneous injection of local anaesthetics (we use trimecaine). Anterior wall of the artery is punctured by a special needle; pulsatile blood flow out from the needle occurs; and a J-shaped guide wire is gently introduced. Needle is withdrawn, and introducer sheath 5F or 6F (4F sheaths are also available, however, CAG with 4F catheters usually offers low-quality images) is inserted using the guide wire. When difficulties occur during the guide wire insertion, operator should never push against resistance, but rather visualize the iliac artery or aorta by small amount of contrast and use the special 'slippery' guide wire with very soft tip. The access site is most frequently femoral artery (usually right), but radial artery approach is increasingly used. Comparison of femoral vs. radial approach is in Table 5.1.

Table 5.1 Comparison of femoral vs. radial approach		
	Femoral artery	Radial artery
Procedure duration	*Shorter*	Longer
Radiation dose	*Lower*	Higher
Support in difficult PCI	*Better*	Worse
Occlusion of the access artery	*Extremely rare (<0.1%)*	3% to 5%
Bleeding complications (large haematoma, pseudoaneurysm, retroperitoneal bleeding)	1% to 3%	*Extremely rare*
Patient comfort	Lower (immobilized few hours after procedure)	*Better (can walk out from the cath-lab)*

Catheters. Most frequently used catheters for CAG are the Judkins shape: left Judkins (JL3, JL4, JL5, JL6—sizes depend on the size of the patient's aorta) and right Judkins (JR3, JR4, JR5, JR6). Second most frequent shape is Amplatz (AL1, AL2, AL3, AR1, AR2). Amplatz catheters require more experience for the manoeuvers; Judkins are more easy to learn. Venous bypass grafts are mostly cannulated by the right Judkins catheters, for left internal mammary artery (LIMA) graft a specially designed catheter is used. Ventriculographic pigtail catheter is used for left ventriculography or aortography.

Techniques to prevent complications. Several precautions have to be strictly followed to avoid potentially fatal complications (stroke, myocardial infarction, etc.).

All catheters and guide wires should be adequately flushed before inserting them into the patient (any—even very small—residual blood clot may serve as a 'triggering nucleus' for the formation of a larger clot when in contact with the patient's blood).

No guide wire/catheter advancement is allowed against resistance. When resistance to catheter advancement occurs, careful fluoroscopic evaluation (including small contrast bolus) should be done to clarify the reason for this resistance.

Free backflow of blood should always be seen before catheter is connected to the stop-cock with contrast and pressure capsule.

First catheter flushing with saline (or heparinized saline) should be done distally to carotid arteries origins (i.e. in descending aorta).

Whenever any potential catheter patency problem (no free backflow of blood, damped pressure curve, etc.) occurs, catheter should be withdrawn down to descending aorta before any attempts to analyse the problem further.

Judkins catheter insertion to the left coronary ostium should be done slowly under the fluoroscopic control to avoid 'fast deep jump-in' to the left main (risk of left main dissection). When this "deep jump-in" occurs, catheter should not be left in such position, but should be slightly withdrawn to avoid contrast injection subintimally.

Cannulation of the right coronary artery (RCA) with the Judkins catheter always requires simultaneous catheter rotation with slight (few centimetres) backward catheter withdrawal.

Smooth pressure curve with typical aortic shape is a good proof that catheter is not pushing against the arterial wall. Thus, watching the aortic pressure curve is very useful during CAG to prevent mechanical complications caused by the catheter.

Meticulous control for any potential air bubbles must be done during the entire procedure. Coronary air embolism may be a serious complication, leading to myocardial infarction or even death (when the amount of air is significant).

Hand injection of a few millilitres of contrast ('test') through the pigtail catheter is recommended before automatic pump is connected and left ventriculography performed. This helps to avoid intramyocardial contrast injection and is absolutely essential in aortic stenosis (where hand injection is usually sufficient to obtain good image, while pump injection may lead to ventricular rupture when too high speed or volume is used).

Post-catheterization care. After uncomplicated elective CAG patients may stay in standard ward (no ECG monitoring is needed) and may be discharged home when the access site is absolutely safe (usually several hours after radial approach and next day after femoral approach). When any complication occurs, patient should be moved to the intensive care unit for closer follow-up and potential treatment. The care for the access site is in the centre of post-catheterization care and is usually done by experienced nurses. The compression of the arterial puncture site should be firm enough to eliminate any potential bleeding, but must not be too firm (neither to eliminate any distal arterial blood flow, nor to obstruct venous return from the extremity). When bleeding occurs, the best solution is to remove the compression completely, press the puncture site manually for several minutes, and then use a new compression binding. The duration of compression depends mostly on the patient's coagulation and blood pressure. For example, elective patients with low blood pressure and no heparin used during the procedure may have compression only for 2 to 3 h (or may even have only 'sandy bag' over the puncture site). On the other hand, patients with hypertension, who received heparin, should have the compression for at least 6 h.

5.4 Coronary angiographic views—angiography of the native coronary arteries

Table 5.2 lists the most frequently used views in CAG.

Figures 5.1 to 5.12 show the coronary angiographic views and anatomy.

CAG remains the most precise method for the evaluation of the entire coronary arterial tree: its anatomy and pathology, and partly also pathophysiology. The examination is invasive and thus the invasive cardiologist is obliged to obtain high-quality images and to visualize all coronary segments and lesions. The cardiologist must be 100% certain about the findings before ending the procedure. When there is any uncertainity due to overlapping structures or low quality of coronary opacification, additional views should be done or more contrast (or larger catheters) should be used.

Table 5.2 The angiographic views (projections) most frequently used in CAG

View	Abbreviation	Angulation (right-left/ cranio-caudal)	Optimal visualization of
Right anterior oblique	RAO	30°/0°	Overall information about the left coronary artery
Right superior oblique	RSO	50°/25°	Left anterior descending (LAD) artery
Right inferior oblique	RIO	30°/−20°	Left circumflex (LCX) artery
Anteroposterior	AP	0°/0°	Left main coronary artery (LMCA)
Cranial	CRAN	0°/30°	LAD + diagonal/ septal branches, RCA bifurcation + posterior descending + right posterolateral
Caudal	CAUD	0°/−30°	LMCA + LCX + obtuse marginal branches
Left anterior oblique	LAO	−30°/0°	RCA
Left superior oblique (LSO; four-chamber)	LSO	−45°/30°	LMCA + LAD + diagonal + left posterolateral (when present)
Left inferior oblique (spider)	LIO	−40°/−30°	LMCA bifurcation + LCX
Left lateral	LL	−90°/0°	LAD + LCX + RCA
Left superior lateral	LSL	−90°/20°	LAD + diagonal
Left inferior lateral	LIL	−90°/−20°	LAD + LCX proximal

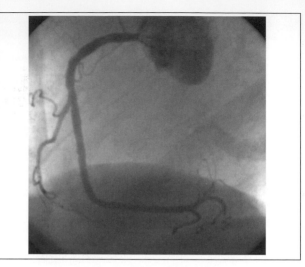

Figure 5.1 The right coronary artery (RCA) in the left lateral (LL) view. The 6F Judkins Right 4 (JR4) catheter is positioned in the coronary ostium and the blood in the artery is fully replaced by the contrast, so that the backflow of contrast to the aortic root is visible. This is the way to obtain high-quality images.
This coronary artery has diffuse, non-obstructive atherosclerotic plaques.

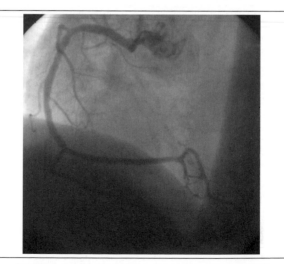

Figure 5.2 RCA in the LSO view. This view allows better assessment of RCA branches than the classical LAO view. Non-obstructive atherosclerotic plaques are visible in the middle segment.

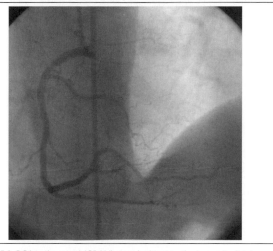

Figure 5.3 RCA in the cranial (CRAN) view. In this view the two main distal branches are best separated: upper (in this case bigger) one is the right poster-olateral artery (ramus posterolateralis dexter), lower one is the posterior descending artery (ramus interventricularis posterior). Diffuse non-obstructive atherosclerotic plaques are visible.

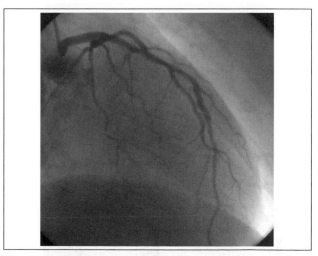

Figure 5.4 Left coronary artery (LCA) in the RAO view. Despite this view is the 'classical' one, it is used less frequently today, because the branches (LAD, LCX, diagonal) are partly overlapping. Superior angulation (RSO) allows better visualiza-tion of LAD and its branches, while inferior angulation (RIO) allows better visualization of LCX and its branches (see Figure 5.5).

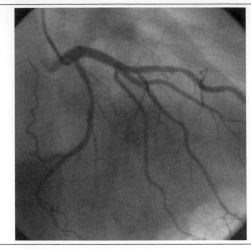

Figure 5.5 LCA in RIO view. A small slightly atherosclerotic LCX (left part of the image) with three very small obtuse marginal branches is visualized. Big diagonal branches (middle) are supplying the lateral wall. LAD (upper branch) has non-obstructive atherosclerotic plaques.

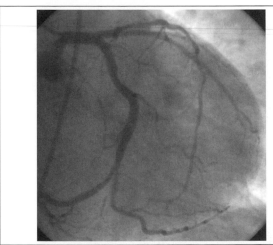

Figure 5.6 LCA in the caudal (CAUD) view in a patient with left dominant type of the coronary tree. Big LCX is supplying the entire intero-postero-lateral wall of the left ventricle (RCA in the left dominant situation supplies only right ventricle). Distal LCX bifurcation gives in LCX dominancy two large branches: posterior descending artery and (left) posterolateral artery. In this case, mild in-stent restenosis is visible in the origins of both these branches.

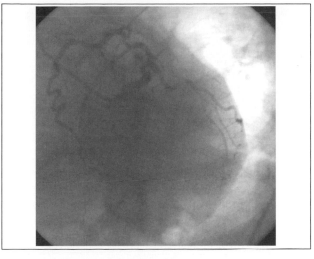

Figure 5.7 LCA in the left inferior oblique (LIO) or 'spider' view. In most patients this is the best view to visualize the LMCA bifurcation. In this case, the LMCA is tortuous, long, and the distal segment is narrowed by cca 40%. A significant (cca 80%) stenosis is visualized on LCX cca 2.5 cm after its origin.

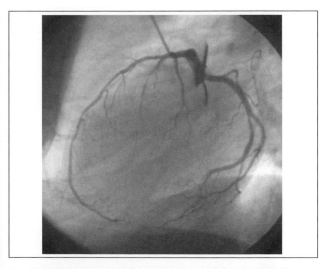

Figure 5.8 LCA in the LL view. The same patient as in Figure 5.6, LAD (left) has diffuse non-obstructive atherosclerotic plaques, dominant LCX has mild in-stent restenosis in the bifurcation.

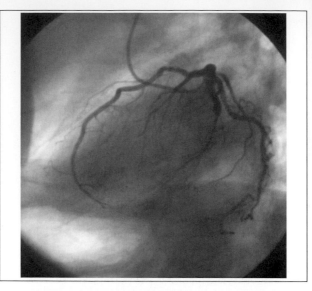

Figure 5.9 LCA in the left inferior lateral (LIL) view.

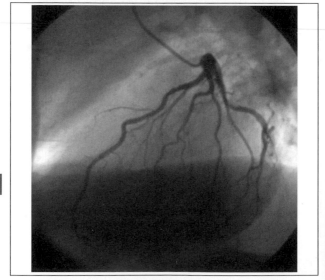

Figure 5.10 LCA in the left superior lateral (LSL) view.

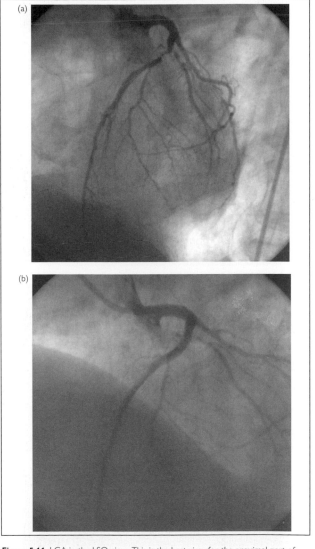

Figure 5.11 LCA in the LSO view. This is the best view for the proximal part of the LMCA and also for LAD bifurcations with its diagonal branches. (a) Cca 80% stenosis of proximal LAD is visualized between the origins of the first and second diagonal branches. Diffuse non-obstructive atherosclerosis is visible in all other branches. (b) Same patient after stent implantation.

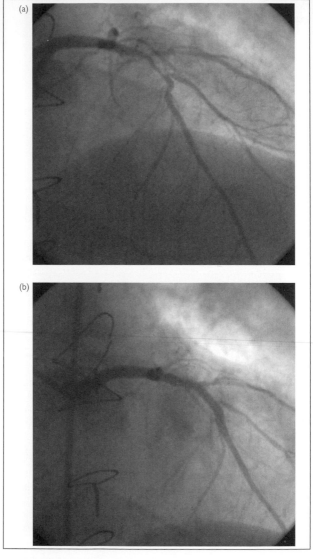

Figure 5.12 LCA in CRAN view. This is the best view (along with RSO) to visualize LAD. (a) proximal cca 70% LAD stenosis is visible between the origin of second and third diagonal branches, both of them having ostial stenoses as well. (b) After stent implantation.

Most frequent 'technical' mistakes leading to low-quality coronary angiogram:

1. Coronary angiogram is done in a pre-specified routine number and sequence of projections, catheters are pulled out and during the images review uncertainty about significance of some of the lesions or filling of some of the branches occurs. (Solution: careful review before pulling out the catheters and performing additional views to visualize the problem better.)

2. Inappropriately thin catheters have been used, which did not allow sufficient volume of contrast at sufficient speed to completely replace the blood in the coronary artery for the few seconds of image recording. Resulting image is weak, grey, and some lesions may be overlooked or the significance of some lesions cannot be assessed correctly. For most coronary arteries, the use of 5F diagnostic catheters provides sufficient image quality, while 4F catheters do not allow this in a substantial number of patients. In patients with high coronary flow (e.g. in left ventricular hypertrophy or with increased cardiac output), even 5F catheters may not provide optimal image quality and 6F should be used. (Solution: avoiding 4F catheters and individual decision between 5F and 6F case by case. Pre-heating of the contrast on the body temperature (37°C).)

3. Image recording is interrupted simultaneously with contrast injection. The resulting images cannot provide sufficient information about the myocardial blush and about the collaterals. (Solution: recording must continue cca 1 to 4 s after the end of contrast injection (until contrast wash out from the myocardium).

As mentioned earlier, the number, sequence, and angulation of the imaging views (projections) should be always individualized. Three projections (usually RAO, LL, and LSO) of the left coronary artery and a single projection (usually LAO) of the right coronary artery may be sufficient in a patient with normal coronary angiogram. On the other hand, more than the mentioned 12 projections may be needed in a patient with complex coronary anatomy and pathology (e.g. left dominant type with multiple complex lesions in all branches). The recording speed most frequently used is 12 to 15 frames/s. Double speed (25 to 30/s) offers higher image quality at the price of increased radiation dose and large storage memory needed. Image size should be between 14 and 17″ (for RAO and LL views 23″ is better).

5.5 **Angiography of coronary bypass grafts**

LIMA bypass graft originates in the native LIMA take off, that is from the inferior wall of the proximal segment of the left subclavian artery, just in its band from its originally cranial course towards the left arm. Selective catheterization is best done by a specific LIMA diagnostic catheter, which is first advanced to the aortic arch, then slowly pulled back while simultaneously rotated. During this manoeuver the tip of the catheter 'jumps' into the proximal left subclavian artery. J-shaped guide wire is advanced through the catheter to the distal subclavian artery, the catheter is then advanced on the guide wire cca 2 to 3 cm distally to the subclavian artery band. Guide wire is removed and small volume of contrast is injected to ascertain the position of the catheter in the subclavian artery. Catheter (with its tip pointing down) is then slowly pulled back and slightly rotated anticlockwise until it fits the LIMA ostium. Image recording is done best with image size 23" in AP and LL (Figure 5.13) projections. It is important to remember that LIMA origin is a specially fragile site, prone to catheter-induced dissections (which may have disastrous consequences due to the importance of the served territory). Thus all the manoeuvers during LIMA examinations should be done very softly and slowly.

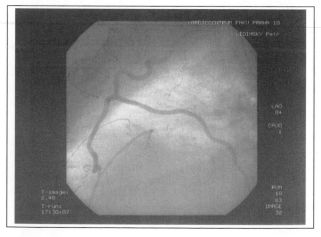

Figure 5.13 The Y-type arterial bypass graft in the LL view. The standard LIMA graft has visible anastomosis on LAD, the free right internal mammary artery (RIMA) graft is going posteroinferiorly and outside the image (right lower corner) is attached to the obtuse marginal branch.

Other arterial grafts (RIMA, radial artery free graft, gastroepiploic artery) are less frequently used and their description is beyond the scope of this pocket book.

Venous bypass grafts originate at the anterior wall of the ascending aorta. Their cannulation is best done in the LL view (Figure 5.14).

Their visualization is usually possible with the same right coronary catheter (mostly Judkins), which was used for the visualization of the right coronary artery. The projections should be selected based on the distal anastomosis: RAO or LL views for venous grafts to LAD, cranial or LSO views for diagonal grafts, RIO, caudal, or LL for obtuse marginal grafts, and LL or LAO for the RCA grafts (Figure 5.15).

It is very important to have the surgical report (with the description of all grafts and their anastomoses) available before the start of CAG. CAG should not finish before the status of all grafts is known. When a venous graft cannot be visualized, it is important that the supply to its territory must be visible either via collaterals or via native coronary artery. Blood supply to all segments of the heart must be known at the end of CAG. Rarely, subclavian artery may be occluded (Figure 5.16) and LIMA visualization is possible only via left radial/brachial artery.

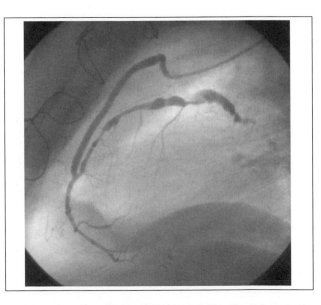

Figure 5.14 Venous bypass graft to LAD in LL view. LAD is diffusely diseased with marked ectasia of the proximal segment with subsequent significant (cca 80%) stenosis. This stenosis is difficult to quantify due to the fact that adjacent segments are severely diseased (so the reference segment is missing).

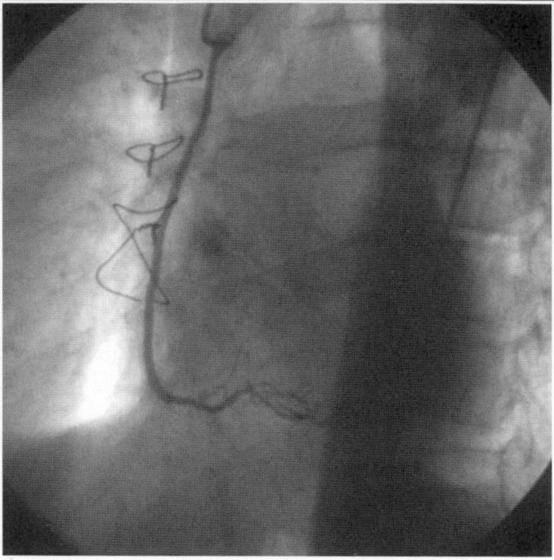

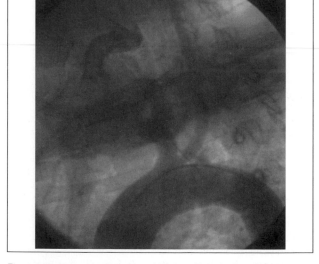

Figure 5.15 Venous graft to RCA (right posterior descending branch) in LAO view.

Figure 5.16 Aortic arch angiography in LAO view. Normal origins of brachio-cephalic trunk and left common carotid artery and proximal occlusion of the left subclavian artery. In this situation, LIMA graft cannot be cannulated via the femoral approach.

5.6 **Most frequent congenital coronary anomalies in adults**

LCX artery origin from the right coronary sinus (or from the proximal segment of the right coronary artery). This is one of the most frequent abnormalities, which usually does not cause symptoms. Only LAD artery (giving its normal diagonal and septal branches) originates from the left coronary sinus. This anomaly can be overlooked when a large diagonal branch of LAD is falsely considered to be a small circumflex. Always, when in the LL view circumflex artery is not visualized, its origin has to be searched in the proximity of the right coronary ostium.

Abnormal origin of the right coronary artery. Right coronary artery may present a challenge for an inexperienced cardiologist, who may spend substantial time and radiation by searching for it when its ostium is not in the typical position within the right coronary sinus. The right coronary origin can be more cranially on the anterior aortic wall (i.e. above the coronary sinuses) or can be in the left coronary sinus. Rarely, the RCA may originate from the pulmonary artery (this is a clear pathology, as far as the supplied myocardium receives blood with low oxygen content).

Coronary fistulae. A congenital communication (an additional branch or a convolute of small branches) may exist between the coronary artery and pulmonary artery, coronary sinus, or any of the cardiac chambers.

5.7 **Evaluation, interpretation, and description of CAG results**

Coronary angiographic main findings must be clear before the catheters are pulled out (as described earlier in details). The evaluation, interpretation, and description should be ideally done immediately after the procedure. In the case of any doubts, opinion of a second invasive cardiologist has to be obtained before writing the final conclusion. The assessment of the lesion severity is highly subjective and even experienced invasive cardiologists may differ by 20% to 30% when they visually evaluate the same lesion for diameter stenosis. The description of a given lesion should be in agreement with the recommendation given—for example revascularization should not be recommended, when the lesion is described as cca 50% diameter stenosis. If the lesion which is borderline (50% to 60%) by its contours has visible irregularities and intraluminal lucencies (complex lesion), its clinical significance is likely to be different from a 50% to 60% lesion with smooth margins and no luminal lucencies.

What should be mentioned in the report:
- Coronary dominant type (right–left–mixed)
- How many major coronary arteries have stenosis >50% (single–double–triple vessel disease, left main disease, no significant stenosis)
- The quantitative description: percent diameter stenosis for all branches with >50% lesions
- In all borderline lesions (40% to 70%), their qualitative description should be added (smooth, concentric, exulcerated, excentric, thrombus-containing, etc.)
- Any bypass grafts or congenital anomalies
- Any collaterals
- The qualitative description: any thrombi, spasms, muscular bridges, intramural calcifications, diffuse 'diabetic-type' involvement, ectasias, aneurysms, emboli, dissections, and so on.
- Treatment recommendation (PCI–bypass grafting–medical therapy).
- The truly quantitative coronary angiography (QCA) is done by computerized automated contour detection. It is used in research protocols, but only rarely used in the routine clinical setting.

5.8 Complications of CAG

The complication rates are low in experienced high volume centres. The risk of complications is increased in the elderly patients, in low body weight patients, in patients with renal failure, heart failure, and of course in patients with acute coronary syndromes. The catheterization procedure itself should be always completely pain-free for the patient. Thus, when the patient starts to describe any pain during or after CAG, the cardiologist should take it always very seriously—it may be the first sign of a serious complication.

Death resulting from CAG is extremely rare (around 0.1% in most series). It may be caused by acute myocardial infarction, stroke, or major arterial dissection or cardiac perforation. Major dissection of the aorta or iliac artery or coronary/cardiac perforation is almost always related to gross catheter manipulations by an inexperienced physician.

Myocardial infarction or stroke can be either iatrogenic (air embolism, catheter thrombus embolism, vascular dissection) or spontaneous (acute thrombosis and/or spasm in a patient with pre-existing critical unstable stenosis). The risk of periprocedural non-fatal infarction or stroke is 0.1% to 0.5%.

Deep venous thrombosis and/or pulmonary embolism is a rare (below 0.1%) consequence of prolonged arterial compression with bed rest after the procedure. Can be prevented by shorter compression times, adequate hydration, and specifically by proper compression on the femoral artery only (not compressing the femoral vein).

Access site bleeding is the most frequent complication (1% to 2% after CAG, 2% to 5% after PCI performed via femoral approach). The risk is increased by heparin dose (especially when the dose is not adequate to patient's body weight, sex, and age) or by combination of several anti-thrombotic drugs. The risk is increased when multiple arterial punctures were needed to cannulate the artery (the final puncture is 'closed' by the sheath, but any previous arterial punctures may leak during/after the procedure). Clearly, the risk is increased with larger catheter (sheath) size. The bleeding risk is substantially smaller with radial artery approach.

Contrast nephropathy. Radiocontrast-induced nephropathy is the third most common cause of in-hospital acute renal failure after hypotension and surgery. Up to 2% to 10% patients after catheterization develop contrast nephropathy. The routine haemodialysis after the administration of contrast media in patients with a reduced renal function did not diminish the rate of complications. The following guidelines for the prevention of contrast nephropathy in patients at high risk were instituted: aggressive hydration before contrast administration, avoidance of exceeding a maximum contrast dose according to the formula *5cc × body weight (kg)/creatinine (mg/dL)*, use of low-osmolar non-ionic contrast; some centres use N-acetylcysteine 600 mg twice per day started on the day before the procedure.

Contrast allergy is very rare with the use of modern contrast agents and is almost always manifested by a skin rash. In our centre, performing cca 3000 coronary angiograms per year, the last serious contrast allergy (i.e. anaphylaxis), was seen six years ago. Old contrast agents used in the past caused this complication more frequently.

Other complications are either extremely rare (e.g. fragmentation of the catheter within patient's body, iatrogenic infection, etc.) or clinically insignificant (e.g. transient arrhythmias caused mechanically by catheter manipulations or during the contrast passage through the coronary artery).

5.9 Other coronary diagnostic techniques: intravascular ultrasound (IVUS), coronary and fractional flow reserve, optical coherence tomography (OCT), angioscopy

IVUS (Figure 5.17a) greatly contributed to the understanding of coronary stent implantation, and to the progress of interventional cardiology as a practical research tool, allowing us to better understand what we are actually doing in the coronary arteries. IVUS precisely describes the stent apposition to the arterial wall, any arterial dissections, and can quantify the lesion severity (and also the PCI result) by measuring vessel cross-sectional area. However, the clinical application of IVUS for routine patient care is questionable—it was never proved in a prospective randomized trial that the use of IVUS improves clinical outcomes.

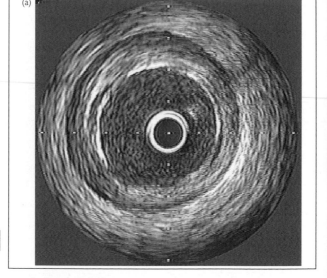

Figure 5.17 Intracoronary ultrasound. (a) Intracoronary imaging (IVUS). The dark black 'hole' in the middle with white sharp margins is the catheter, surrounded by low echo density (black colour) arterial lumen and layers of arterial wall.

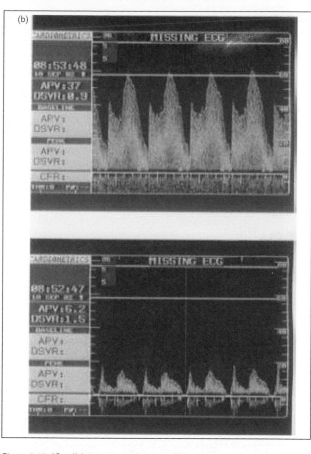

Figure 5.17 (*Contd.*) Intracoronary ultrasound. (b) Intracoronary Doppler—coronary flow reserve measurement. Resting flow velocity 6.2 cm/s (lower part) and hyperemic (after papaverine) flow velocity 37 cm/s (upper image). Calculated coronary flow reserve is 37/6.2 = 5.96.

Coronary reserve can be measured by several methods: computerized CAG (myocardial flow reserve, least precise), intracoronary Doppler (coronary flow reserve, more precise—Figure 5.17b) or intracoronary tip-manometer (coronary fractional flow reserve, most precise). The normal physiologic values of coronary reserve are 4 to 10, which means that a normal coronary artery is capable to increase the flow 4 to 10 times in response to the increase of myocardial oxygen consumption (e.g. during maximal exercise). Exercise during CAG is not optimal, thus pharmacologic stimuli (adenosine, papaverine [not licensed in the UK]) are usually used to test the coronary reserve. These methods have very interesting research and physiologic implications; however, they are not really needed for clinical decision making. Their description is beyond the scope of this pocket book.

OCT is a young method, providing more detailed visualization of the coronary artery lumen and intima. It is less capable to assess the arterial wall. Its role in clinical practice has yet to be established.

Angioscopy allows direct visualization of the coronary lumen on a principle similar to any endoscopy. Its use is largely limited by the need to occlude the artery by a balloon and replace the blood by saline to visualize the lumen. It remains thus only a research tool.

Key reading

Baim D. Coronary angiography. In: *Grossman's Cardiac Catheterization, Angiography and Intervention*, Seventh edition, edited by Baim D. Lippincott Williams & Wilkins, Philadelphia, 2006.

Balter S, Baim DS. Cineangiographic imaging, radiation safety and contrast agents. In: *Grossman's Cardiac Catheterization, Angiography and Intervention*, Seventh edition, edited by Baim D. Lippincott Williams & Wilkins, Philadelphia, 2006.

Bassand JP, Hamm CV, Ardissino D et al. ESC Guidelines for the diagnosis and treatment of non-ST-segment elevation acute coronary syndromes. *Eur Heart J* 2007; **28**: 1598–660.

Boden WE, O'Rourke RA, Teo KK et al. COURAGE Trial Research Group. Optimal medical therapy with or without PCI for stable coronary disease. *N Engl J Med* 2007; **356**: 1503–16.

Fox K, Alonso Garcia MA, Ardissino D et al. ESC Guidelines for the management of stable angina pectoris. *Eur Heart J* 2006; **27**: 1341–81.

Hueb W, Lopes NH, Gersh BJ et al. Five-year follow-up of the Medicine, Angioplasty or Surgery Study (MASS II). *Circulation* 2007; **115**: 1082–9.

Kandzari DE, Rebeiz AG, Wang A et al. Contrast nephropathy: an evidence-based approach to prevention. *Am J Cardiovasc Drugs* 2003; **3**(6): 395–405.

Kefer JM, Hanet CE, Boitte S. Meta-analysis of randomized clinical trials on the usefulness of acetylcysteine for prevention of contrast nephropathy. *Am J Cardiol* 2003; **92**(12): 1454–8.

Silber S, Albertsson P, Fernandez-Aviles F et al. ESC Guidelines for percutaneous coronary interventions. *Eur Heart J* 2005; **26**: 804–47.

Vogt B, Ferrari P, Schonholzer C et al. Prophylactic hemodialysis after radiocontrast media in patients with renal insufficiency is potentially harmful. *Am J Med* 2001; **111**(9): 692–8.

Widimsky P, Motovska Z, Simek S et al.; Aschermann M on behalf of the PRAGUE-8 trial Investigators. Clopidogrel pre-treatment in stable angina: for all patients >6 h before elective coronary angiography or only for angiographically selected patients a few minutes before PCI? A randomized multicentre trial PRAGUE-8. *Eur Heart J* 2008; **29**: 1495–503.

Chapter 6

Left ventricular angiography and other angiocardiographic techniques

Giuseppe De Luca, Elena Franchi, Petr Widimsky, Harry Suryapranata

Key points

- Left ventriculography (LVG) provides information about left ventricular (LV) function, mitral regurgitation, ventricular septal defect, hypertrophic cardiomyopathy, and intraventricular thrombus.
- Aortography remains the standard for pre-operative assessment of thoracic aorta aneurysms, aortic regurgitation, coarctation, or other congenital anomalies, to visualize questionable coronary bypass grafts and to assess proximal segments of aortic branches.
- Pulmonary angiography is used for the diagnosis of pulmonary embolism, arteriovenous malformation, and anomalous pulmonary venous return.
- The cardiologist may decide to add angiography of the carotid, renal, or pelvic arteries on top of coronary angiography (CAG) to diagnose pathologies of these arteries.

6.1 LVG

LVG may provide information about global LV function and segmental wall motion, mitral regurgitation, ventricular septal defect, hypertrophic cardiomyopathy, intraventricular thrombus, and so on. Long image registration (after the contrast exits the LV) with simultaneous cath-lab table motion may allow thoracic aorta visualization from a single contrast injection.

Ventriculographic catheters should have multiple side holes and 6F lumen allows good LV opacification. The most frequently used is the angled Judkins pigtail catheter.

Injection site, rate, and volume. The optimal catheter position is the midcavity. When midcavity position produces extrasystoles, LV inflow tract position may be used, but this is at the cost of artificial mitral regurgitation in some patients. When catheter tip is located in the apex, the injection rate should be decreased to only 10 mL/s. Power injectors allow selecting the volume and the rate of contrast delivery. This selection should be based on the following variables:

• Catheter type and size
• LV size
• Cardiac output (LV stroke volume + heart rate)
• Presence/absence of LV outflow obstruction.

The injection should last for 3 s; the volume injected is mostly 30 to 36 mL, with a rate of 10 to 12 mL/s. Higher volume and rate may be used in high cardiac output situations or when LV cavity is large. Smaller volumes and rates should be used for small ventricles and especially in aortic stenosis or other LV outflow obstruction situations. It is absolutely essential to perform appropriate precautions in filling and firing the power injector to prevent air embolism.

Technique, projections. It is useful to perform a small (test) contrast injection by hand before the power injector is connected to the catheter. This allows verifying of the catheter position and gives some idea about the rate of contrast wash out from the LV allowing the power injector individualized settings. Prior to performing the ventriculography, the physician should confirm that the injector syringe is filled with contrast, free of air, contrast/blood interface is seen, and the syringe is oriented 'nose-down'. The physician should grasp the catheter to be able to pull it back immediately when myocardial staining or other events develop during the injection. The 30° RAO projection is most frequently used to analyse global and regional LV function and mitral regurgitation. LSO 60°/20° projection is used to visualize the septum and lateral wall and aortic valve morphology. Most CAGs are done at recording speed 12 to 15 frames/s; LVG should be done at 25 to 30 frames/s rate.

Analysis and description of LVG. Only a normal (sinus) beat following previous normal beat should be used for analysis. Regional wall motion is graded as hyper-, normo-, hypo-, a- or dyskinetic. Global LV ejection fraction, end-diastolic and end-systolic volumes (Table 6.1) are calculated by the area–length method after appropriate system calibration.

Table 6.1 Normal left ventricular angiographic values	
LV end-diastolic volume index	50–90 mL/m^2
LV end-systolic volume index	13–35 mL/m^2
LV ejection fraction	0.55–0.75

Mitral regurgitation is detected by contrast appearance in the left atrial cavity and should be semiquantified into four grades:

- 1+ (mild: contrast enters left atrium during systole but clears with each beat)
- 2+ (medium: contrast does not clear with each beat, is less dense than left ventricle, see Figure 1.6)
- 3+ (moderate: opacification of left atrium is equal to that of left ventricle)
- 4+ (severe: opacification of the left atrium is greater than that of the LV, or the presence of contrast in pulmonary veins).

Complications of LVG. Ventricular arrhythmias or fascicular block are usually transient and benign. Extrasystoles alter the LV wall motion and modify mitral regurgitation. Severe complications (myocardial contrast staining, LV perforation or systemic embolism) are rare, but may be fatal.

6.2 Thoracic aortography

Aortography remains the gold standard for the pre-operative assessment of thoracic aorta aneurysms, aortic regurgitation, coarctation, or other congenital anomalies, to visualize questionable coronary bypass grafts, to assess proximal segments of aortic branches, and so on. The pigtail catheter should be positioned just above the sinus of Valsalva and 40 to 60 mL of contrast should be injected by the pump at the rate of 20 mL/s and recording speed of 12 to 15 frames/s. Left anterior oblique (LAO) view is generally used.

Aortic regurgitation is quantified as:

- 1+ (mild: contrast enters left ventricle during diastole and clears with each beat)
- 2+ (medium: contrast opacification of the left ventricle does not clear with each beat and is less dense than ascending aorta)
- 3+ (moderate: opacification of the left ventricle is more than that of the aorta, see Figure 1.7)
- 4+ (severe: opacification of the left ventricle is greater than that of the aorta, or the left ventricle is opacified in one diastolic filling period).

6.3 **Pulmonary angiography**

Pulmonary angiography remains the gold standard for the diagnosis of pulmonary embolism, arteriovenous malformation, anomalous pulmonary venous return, and so on. For more details see Section 4.8.

6.4 **Angiography of carotid, renal, and peripheral arteries**

The peripheral angiography is usually not performed by a cardiologist (rather by a radiologist or angiologist) and is thus beyond the scope of this book. However, occasionally the cardiologist may decide to add angiography of the carotid, renal, or pelvic arteries on top of CAG. The information about carotid arteries may be requested by cardiac surgeons as part of the pre-operative assessment before cardiac surgery of the patient with carotid murmur, recent stroke, or carotid stenosis described by ultrasound. Renal angiography may be done in a patient (undergoing elective CAG) with exceptionally severe refractory hypertension to assess potential renal artery stenosis. Local injection (partial) iliac angiography is frequently done, when cardiologist is facing difficulties to pass the sheath, guide wire, or catheter from the femoral artery to aorta. Anteroposterior view is usually sufficient for renal angiography and local iliac angiography, while multiple (A-P, LL, oblique) views are preferred for carotid angiography.

Key reading

Baim DS. Cardiac ventriculography. In: *Grossman's Cardiac Catheterization, Angiography and Intervention*, edited by Baim DS. Lippincott Williams & Wilkins, Philadelphia, 2006, pp. 222–33.

Croft CH, Lipscomb K, Mathis K *et al.* Limitations of qualitative angiographic grading in aortic or mitral regurgitation. *Am J Cardiol* 1984; **53**: 1593–8.

Jaff MR, MacNeill BD, Rosenfield K. Angiography of the aorta and peripheral arteries. In: *Grossman's Cardiac Catheterization, Angiography and Intervention*, edited by Baim DS. Lippincott Williams & Wilkins, Philadelphia, 2006, pp. 254–79.

Chapter 7

PCI techniques

Giuseppe De Luca, Petr Widimsky,
Harry Suryapranata

> ## Key points
>
> - Material selection and intervention technique are
>   important factors for the procedural success, especially
>   in the high risk subjects.
> - The clinical judgement (based on the knowledge of
>   guidelines) must precede the indication in order to
>   maximize the patient's clinical benefit based on available
>   modern percutaneous coronary intervention (PCI)
>   techniques.
> - Attention should be paid to prevent arterial access site
>   complications and contrast-induced nephropathy (CIN).

The advances in PCI materials (especially stents) and techniques made
it technically feasible to perform a PCI in the vast majority of coronary
lesions (examples include bifurcation lesions, left main lesions, chronic
total occlusions (CTO), multivessel interventions, etc.). The major
challenge in interventional cardiology today is not a technical one, but
rather the opposite: some interventional cardiologists are treating the
coronary lesions and not the patient. A typical example is CTO: PCI is
technically feasible, but the clinical benefit has yet to be proven.
Patient clinical benefit (and not the demonstration of doctor's skills)
must be a priority. When this is kept in mind, the wise use of the
described techniques may be of great help to the patients.

7.1 Material selection

1. Sheaths—Sheath length: long sheaths (24 cm) provide better
   support especially in the case of tortuous iliac vessels, and
   they also better protect these vessels against any potential
   damage during material exchange. Sheath diameter: 5F or
   6F sizes are used for most PCI procedures.
2. Guiding catheters—In addition to serving as a route for
   contrast and materials, catheters should provide a good
   support to cross coronary lesions. The 'pushing balance'

between good support and potential coronary damage (from aggressive, deep intubation) is crucial. When deep coronary artery intubation is needed for the lesion crossing, the guiding catheter must be always 'released' (slightly drawn back) before the balloon (stent) inflation.

3. Guiding catheter size—6F catheters (or 5F for simple procedures) are the standard, since they allow deep engagement, restriction of contrast use, and allow radial approach with the possibility to perform kissing with two monorail balloons. 7F catheters are used for double stenting technique in bifurcations (Crush, V stenting), CTO (stronger support, allowing the use of two over-the-wire (OTW) balloons for parallel wire approach). 8F catheters are needed in case of atherectomy, rotablation (>2.0), intravascular ultrasound (IVUS)-guided CTO recanalization.

4. Guiding catheter shape—The selection of a specific shape is generally based on ascending aorta dimension, coronary ostium location, length of left main, radial or femoral access, and the vessel to be engaged. Judkins catheters are the standard: smaller catheters selectively engage left descending coronary artery, whereas longer left catheters selectively engage circumflex artery, providing a better support. Amplatz catheters provide better support by a deeper coronary intubation at the price of slightly higher risk of coronary dissection. Left Amplatz catheters may be preferred in case of long left main, dilated ascending aorta, and lesions located in circumflex artery, as well as for right coronary artery (RCA) in case of anterior ostium origin. The choice of catheters is also based on the take-off of the artery. JR should be preferred in case of transverse take-off, whereas Hockey-stick or Amplatz catheters may be additionally considered in case of superior take-off, and the multipurpose catheter in case of inferior take-off. XB guiding catheter is also an excellent catheter for extra support.

5. Intracoronary guidewires—In addition to floppy guide wires for routine use (High torque Floppy, BMW Universal, ATW Cordis, Runthrough, etc.), several additional wires have been recommended for use in specific lesions and difficult anatomy. In tortuous vessels hydrophilic guide wires (Choice PT, Whispers, PT2) should be preferred, whereas in chronic occlusions stiffer wires with better support should be considered (Cross-IT, Miracle, Asahi, Shinobi, etc.). Gentle manipulation of the guide wires is mandatory especially in chronic occlusion and in distal positioning of hydrophilic or stiffer wires, due to the higher risk of coronary perforation.

6. Angioplasty balloons—Monorail balloons (with lateral wire exit cca 20 to 30 cm from the balloon/stent distal tip) are the standard in routine PCI. OTW balloons (with guide wire within the central balloon/stent lumen along the shaft length) may be useful in chronic or acute total occlusion (advantages: better crossing support, possibility of local contrast or drug delivery). The use of compliant vs. non-compliant balloons is a matter of debate. Non-compliant balloons (only when their size is properly selected!) are better for stent optimization, especially in the era of drug-eluting stents (DES). Compliant balloons allow better balloon (stent) sizing in wider range to fit the coronary artery size (e.g. a 3.0 mm balloon may be dilated up to 3.4 mm). The selection (type, size, and length) of balloons should be based on coronary anatomy and the extent of the disease. Balloon predilatation may help to cross the lesion and to choose the appropriate stent size.

7. Stents.

The stent type—All coronary stents today are balloon-expandable, that is they are delivered on a deflated angioplasty balloon to the lesion and implanted by the balloon inflation. The final stent expansion luminal diameter is predicted by two factors: the selected stent size (diameter) and the final balloon inflation pressure. Several metallic materials (stainless steel, cobalt chromium, etc.) are used for bare metal stents (BMS). The advantage is relatively fast (within ~3 weeks) endothelial overgrowth over the stent struts, allowing safe clopidogrel discontinuation after 4 weeks. DES have more complex structure, where not only mechanical (as in BMS), but also chemical/pharmaceutical/biological characteristics play an important role. Main DES advantage is the lower risk of restenosis (due to the decreased neointimal hyperplasia), main disadvantage is the need for longer (at least 6 to 12 months) use of clopidogrel (stent thrombosis risk when clopidogrel is discontinued prematurely). The new generation of DES (reabsorbable polymers, shortened drug elution, biodegradable stents) favours complete re-endothelization and may reduce the risk of late in-stent thrombosis. ESC guidelines recommendation for DES and the full list of currently available DES are reported in Table 7.1. Although larger benefits might be expected in high-risk lesions and patients, due to the fear of late in-stent thrombosis, DES are recommended in specific subsets of lesions and patients (with high risk for restenosis) where evidence of safety and benefits have been already accumulated.

The stent size—Appropriate selection of stent size is the key for success of PCI. Stent diameter (usually between 2.5 and 5.0 mm) should be selected according to the coronary artery healthy segment

Table 7.1 ESC guidelines (2005) recommendations for the use of DES in *de novo* lesions of native coronary arteries and the list of currently (2008) available DES

DES	Indication	Recommendation/evidence	Randomized studies for levels A or B
Cypher stent	*De novo* lesions in native vessels according to the inclusion criteria	IB	SIRIUS
Taxus stent	*De novo* lesions in native vessels according to the inclusion criteria	IB	TAXUS-IV
Taxus stent	*De novo* long lesions in native vessels according to the inclusion criteria	IB	TAXUS-VI

Currently (2008) available DES in Europe

Stent name	Eluted drug	Manufacturer	Randomized trials/registries
Cypher	Sirolimus	Cordis/Johnson & Johnson	RAVEL, SIRIUS, DIABETES, BASKET
Taxus Liberté	Paclitaxel	Boston Scientific	TAXUS, BASKET, COREA-TAXUS,
Promus	Everolimus	Boston Scientific	ABSOLUTE
Xience V	Everolimus	Abbott	SPIRIT, FUTURE
Endeavor	Zotarolimus	Medtronic	ENDEAVOR, PRISON
Endeavor® Resolute	Zotarolimus	Medtronic	RESOLUTE
Costar II	Paclitaxel	Conor Medsystems	COSTAR, ABSOLUTE
Axxion	Paclitaxel	Occam/Biosensors	EAGLE
BioMatrix	Biolimus	Biosensors	STEALTH
Infinnium	Paclitaxel	Sahajanad Medical	SIMPLE
Genous	Antibody that captures patient's own endothelial progenitor cells	OrbusNeich	TRAIS trial, HEALING registry
JanusFlex	Tacrolimus	Sorin Biomedica	CORPAL

diameter, and in case of doubts (between two stent sizes, e.g. 3.0 or 3.5 mm), the slightly larger size should be taken (e.g. 3.5 mm). The use of undersized stent (e.g. 3.0 mm stent into a coronary artery with 3.2 to 3.5 mm diameter) increases the risk of stent thrombosis or restenosis (see below). The use of an oversized stent (e.g. 4.0 mm stent into 3.2 to 3.5 mm artery) may cause coronary dissection. Stent length (usually between 8 and 38 mm) should be selected to cover the entire diseased segment or to cover vessel tortuosity distal or proximal to target lesion.

The number of stents
Ideal PCI is performed with only one stent implantation into one coronary artery. The more stents are implanted into one artery, the higher the risk of restenosis or stent thrombosis.

Optimal stent deployment
Stent must be apposed perfectly to the intimal surface, without any spaces left between the stent struts and the endothelium. Any malapposition may cause future stent thrombosis or may facilitate neointimal growth (restenosis). Ideal angiographic result of stent implantation is mild 'negative residual stenosis', that is the diameter of the stented segment is ~10% larger than in the adjacent segments, without any dissection. High pressure inflations are generally used for stent deployment. However, stent size selection is more important than inflation pressure (e.g. an undersized stent cannot be optimally implanted in a larger artery even with the highest possible pressure).

7.2 **PCI technique**

7.2.1 **Elective/ad-hoc PCI in chronic stable angina**
For details see Chapter 8.

7.2.2 **PCI in evolving acute myocardial infarction**
For details see Chapter 9.

7.2.3 **CTO**
CTOs have the lowest technical success rates with PCI. The rationale for recanalization is to improve long-term outcomes, left ventricular ejection fraction (LVEF), electrical stability of myocardium, and tolerance for future coronary events. However, none of these potential benefits have been proven in randomized clinical trials. Therefore, PCI attempt on CTO is one of the most difficult decision to make (time-consuming and technically demanding procedure with lower success rates and more radiation vs. questionable clinical benefit). The ESC guidelines indication for PCI in CTO is IIa C.

The chance for successful recanalization depends on the length of occluded lesion, presence of a tapered stump, origin of a side branch at occlusion site, vessel or lesion tortuosity and calcification, presence of antegrade flow, ostial occlusion, and bridging collaterals.

PCI Techniques for CTO. The classic technique is based on the optimal guiding catheter support, stiffer (hydrophilic) guide wire selection and small size OTW balloon for CTO crossing. OTW technique (Figure 7.1) is safer (allows distal contrast injection before the first balloon inflation—Figure 7.1b) and provides better support when compared with monorail (rapid exchange) technique. Multiple novel PCI techniques have been developed to improve CTO recanalization success rates, but their real place in clinical practice has yet to be defined: balloon anchoring, parallel wire technique, seesaw technique, subintimal tracking and reentry (STAR) technique, retrograde approach, IVUS-guided technique.

In the vast majority of cases (90%), unsuccessful PCI for CTO is due to inability to pass the wire. Therefore, growing attention has been directed towards improvement in CTO crossing.

Guide wires. Hydrophilic wires move more easily through soft tissue, providing improved manoeuverability in tortuous vessels and around sharp bends. However, the hydrophilicity also makes it easier to pass into false lumens or small side branches, which may increase the risk of perforation. The Steer-It™ (Cordis, Miami Lakes, FL) deflecting tip guide wire makes it possible to change the guide wire tip angle and thereby improve the chances of engaging difficult take-off angles, negotiating around tortuous bends, and steering away from dissection planes. However, this device has not been approved for use in CTOs.

Adjunct devices. The Tornus® catheter (Asahi Intec, Japan) is a novel OTW stainless steel penetration catheter. The Venture™ Wire Control Catheter (St. Jude Medical, Inc, St. Paul, MN) is a support catheter that also provides steering control through a deflectable tip. The Crosser™ system (FlowCardia, Inc., Sunnyvale, CA) uses vibration energy (20 kHz ultrasound) transmitted through the tip to facilitate mechanical recanalization. *Lumen Reentry Devices* (Pioneer® catheter—Medtronic, Outback® catheter or Frontrunner® XP CTO Catheter—LuMend) employ different technologies to return guide wires into the true lumen after they have created a dissection plane.

Improving long-term success: DES. Several randomized trials have shown that restenosis rate after CTO angioplasty is 32% to 55%. DES may improve the outcomes in these patients.

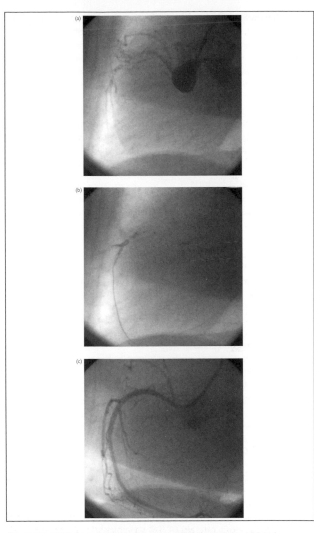

Figure 7.1 CTO recanalization by the classical OTW technique. (a) Initial angiogram of the RCA in LL view showing the proximal chronic RCA occlusion with bridging collaterals faintly opacifying RCA mid-segment. (b) The balloon was advanced through an Amplatz Right 2 guiding catheter over the 300 cm intracoronary wire to the occlusion site, wire was removed and contrast was injected via the central lumen of the OTW balloon. Contrast filling of the distal RCA lumen is a prove for the good position of the balloon, which can be (after re-introduction of the guide wire distally) now safely inflated. (c) Final result after stent placement.

7.2.4 **Multivessel PCI**

Multivessel PCI is technically feasible and routinely performed in most centres. The decision to perform multivessel PCI should be based on the solid assessment of the best patient's interest—that is, to consider surgical revascularization or medical therapy as alternatives. It was never proved whether PCI of all >50% lesions is superior to PCI of only one or two most critical (ischemia-induced) lesions. Similarly, in a patient with acute coronary syndrome (ACS), PCI of the culprit lesion only may be clinically sufficient, while many centres routinely perform PCI of other significant lesions even when it is not known at the time of ACS whether these lesions will ever cause any clinical problems to the patient. Randomized trials on this question are ongoing.

7.2.5 **Bifurcation lesions**

The bifurcation PCI is technically more challenging and has the highest rates of restenosis, particularly when a multiple stent approach is used. Four techniques may be used to treat bifurcation lesions, depending on the diameter of the target segments.

1. *Provisional stenting* is preferred when the side branch is significantly smaller than the main branch.
2. *Kissing stenting* is preferred when both distal branches have similar (or large) diameter and the proximal segment is large enough to accommodate two stents. An 8F guiding catheter is used to precisely align two stents juxtaposed to each other. The stents are inflated simultaneously to create a new carina at the distal bifurcation.
3. *T-Stenting* is less commonly used because of higher restenosis rates. Final kissing balloon inflations may be performed to obtain optimal stent apposition.
4. *Crush stenting* is preferred when there is significant disease in the proximal segment but the artery is not large enough to accommodate two fully expanded stents. Final kissing balloon inflations should be performed to obtain optimal stent apposition and decrease the risk of restenosis or thrombosis.

7.2.6 **Left main coronary artery (LMCA)**

PCI in a (bypass graft) protected LMCA can be regarded as PCI of the proximal segment of LAD or LCX. PCI in unprotected LMCA carries higher acute (dissection, thrombosis) and long-term (restenosis, stent thrombosis) risk due to the amount of myocardium at risk. Enthusiasm for the benefit of DES has encouraged some to advocate its use in LMCA stenosis, for which coronary artery bypass grafting (CABG) is traditionally regarded as the standard of care because of durable survival advantage. To date only one small randomized trial (LEMANS trial) for unprotected LMCA has been reported. MACE at 1 yr was similar in the two groups, while 15% of the PCI group required further PCI or CABG. The SYNTAX trial showed that for isolated LMCA stenosis PCI can be an alternative to CABG, while in LMCA stenosis with MVD, CABG is still the preferred option.

7.2.7 Saphenous vein grafts (SVG)

PCI in SVG has a specific risk of distal embolization of the soft plaques (debris) from the graft to the distal native coronary artery, resulting in slow-flow or no-flow phenomenon, which is difficult to treat and may result in a periprocedural myocardial infarction. Distal protection devices are recommended in this setting. The stent size selection should reflect the larger diameter of the original saphenous vein (in general, larger stents are used for SVG).

7.2.8 Debulking techniques

The debulking techniques (coronary atherectomy, rotablation, laser angioplasty, etc.) were not shown to provide better results when compared with balloon dilatation + stent, but they may cause more complications and restenoses. Thus, they are largely abandoned today.

7.3 Restenosis

Restenosis is caused by a slow progression of neointimal growth. It takes 1 to 6 months before full restenosis develops. Angiographic restenosis was described in >30% after balloon angioplasty, in 15% to 20% after BMS and in 5% to 10% of DES implantation. PCI for restenosis is usually done as 'DES into BMS' implantation or as larger balloon dilatation of the original stent. DES is certainly the best prevention and treatment of restenosis, but the risk of another restenosis remains. The potential benefit of a newly developed drug-eluting balloon for in-stent restenosis has recently been reported. Restenosis is considered 'a benign iatrogenic disorder': reflecting its usually benign course (either clinically silent or with slow return of angina) and its iatrogenic cause (many restenoses are caused by suboptimal result of the original PCI procedure, stent undersizing, etc.).

7.4 Arterial access for PCI

Transfemoral access is most routinely used due to its technical simplicity, whereas transradial access is gaining popularity due to its lower complication profile. Less entry site complications but a lower rate of procedural success, due to its higher technical requirement, have been observed with transradial as compared to transfemoral access in a recent meta-analysis. The incidence of femoral vascular complications after PCI is reported to be around 2% to 6%, including haematoma, pseudo-aneurysm, arteriovenous (AV) fistula formation, lower limb ischaemia, femoral artery infection, and retroperitoneal bleeding.

Femoral haematoma usually resolves with time and does not require specific therapy. Pseudo-aneurysms and AV fistulas usually resolve with compression, which can be performed with or without ultrasound guidance. Vascular surgical repair is rarely required. Retroperitoneal bleeding is a serious complication caused by a high puncture site above the inguinal ligament. The incidence of retroperitoneal bleeding after PCI is reported to be <0.5%.

Femoral access site infection is a rare but increasingly complex problem due to the increasing use of artery closure devices. The two commonly used devices are Perclose (Abbott Laboratories, Abbott Park, IL, USA), a suture-based device, and Angioseal (St. Jude Medical, St. Paul, MN, USA), a collagen plug device. Their use significantly improved patient's comfort, with early post-PCI mobilization. However, use of closure devices has not been shown to reduce the risk of access site complications, but may increase the risk of access site infection.

Radial artery access is in general more comfortable for the patient and carries a lower risk of bleeding complications. Loss of the radial pulse may occur, but usually this does not cause hand ischaemia if adequate collateral circulation from the ulnar artery could be demonstrated with Allen's test before the procedure.

7.5 **Radiographic contrast agents for PCI**

Contrast media can be categorized according to osmolarity (high-osmolar contrast media (HOCM) ~2000 mOsmol/kg, low-osmolar contrast media (LOCM) 600 to 800 mOsmol/kg, and iso-osmolar contrast media (IOCM) 290 mOsmol/kg). Red blood cell deformation, systemic vasodilation, intrarenal vasoconstriction, and renal tubular toxicity may potentially be induced by contrast agents with osmolarity greater than that of blood. Iso-osmolar contrast agent, iodixanol, has been shown to have the lowest risk for CIN.

Volume of contrast. Numerous studies have shown that the volume of contrast medium is a risk factor for contrast-induced renal failure. As a general rule, the volume of contrast used should not exceed twice the baseline level of eGFR in millilitres.

Prevention of CIN. Several randomized trials have shown that isotonic fluid administration (0.9% saline solution at 1 mL/kg/h) 12 h before and after angiography ± PCI reduces CIN. Acetylcysteine may provide additional benefits. Key points in the prevention of CIN are:

1. Identification of high-risk patients (evaluation of creatinine clearance)
2. Hydration (with or without) acetylcysteine
3. Use of isosmolar contrast
4. Use of limited contrast volume.

Key reading

Agostoni P, Biondi-Zoccai GG, de Benedictis ML et al. Radial versus femoral approach for percutaneous coronary diagnostic and interventional procedures; systematic overview and meta-analysis of randomized trials. J Am Coll Cardiol 2004; **44**: 349–56.

Aspelin P, Aubry P, Fransson SG et al. Nephrotoxic effects in high-risk patients undergoing angiography. N Engl J Med 2003; **348**: 491–9.

Brodie BR. Adjunctive balloon postdilatation after stent deployment: is it still necessary with drug-eluting stents? J Interv Cardiol 2006; **19**: 43–50.

Davidson C, Stacul F, McCullough PA et al. Contrast medium use. Am J Cardiol 2006; **98**: 42K–58K.

De Luca G, Stone GW, Suryapranata H et al. Efficacy and safety of drug-eluting stents in ST-segment elevation myocardial infarction: a meta-analysis of randomized trials. Int J Cardiol, 2 April 2008 [Epub ahead of print].

Lakovou I, Schmidt T, Bonizzoni E et al. Incidence, predictors, and outcome of thrombosis after successful implantation of drug-eluting stents. JAMA 2005; **293**(17): 2126–30.

Laskey WK, Jenkins C, Selzer F et al. NHLBI Dynamic Registry Investigators Volume-to-creatinine clearance ratio: a pharmacokinetically based risk factor for prediction of early creatinine increase after percutaneous coronary intervention. J Am Coll Cardiol 2007; **50**: 584–90.

Morice MC, Serruys PW, Sousa JE et al. RAVEL Study Group. Randomized Study with the Sirolimus-Coated Bx Velocity Balloon-Expandable Stent in the Treatment of Patients with de Novo Native Coronary Artery Lesions. A randomized comparison of a sirolimus-eluting stent with a standard stent for coronary revascularization. N Engl J Med 2002; **346**(23): 1773–80.

Moses JW, Leon MB, Popma JJ et al. SIRIUS Investigators. Sirolimus-eluting stents versus standard stents in patients with stenosis in a native coronary artery. N Engl J Med 2003; **349**(14): 1315–23.

Rudnick MR, Goldfarb S, Wexler L et al. The Iohexol Cooperative study, Nephrotoxicity of ionic and nonionic contrast media in 1196 patients: a randomized trial. Kidney Int 1995; **47**: 254–61.

Silber S, Albertsson P, Aviles FF *et al.* Guidelines for percutaneous coronary interventions: the task force for percutaneous coronary interventions of the European Society of Cardiology. *Eur Heart J* 2005; **26**: 804–47

Solomon R. The role of osmolality in the incidence of contrast-induced nephropathy: a systematic review of angiographic contrast media in high risk patients. *Kidney Int* 2005; **68**: 2256–63.

Stettler C, Wandel S, Allemann S *et al.* Outcomes associated with drug-eluting and bare-metal stents: a collaborative network meta-analysis. *Lancet* 2007; **370**(9591): 937–48.

Stone GW, Ellis SG, Cannon L *et al.*; TAXUS V Investigators. Comparison of a polymer-based paclitaxel-eluting stent with a bare metal stent in patients with complex coronary artery disease: a randomized controlled trial. *JAMA* 2005; **294**(10): 1215–23.

Chapter 8

PCI for chronic stable coronary artery disease

Giuseppe De Luca, Elena Franchi,
Harry Suryapranata

> **Key points**
>
> - Percutaneous coronary intervention (PCI) in chronic
>   stable patients is indicated when symptoms are difficult
>   to control despite optimal medical therapy, when large
>   ischemic area and the lesions are suitable for a
>   percutaneous approach.
> - PCI in chronic stable patients does not decrease the risk
>   of death or myocardial infarction in stable patients.

The survival rate of patients with chronic stable coronary artery
disease (CAD) depends on left ventricular (LV) function and on the
number of diseased vessels. Involvement of the left main coronary
artery (LMCA) or proximal left anterior descending artery (LAD)
increases the risk.

According to the ESC guidelines on stable angina, coronary
angiography is recommended for diagnostic purposes or for risk
stratification (Table 8.1).

8.1 Treatment of stable CAD

Any treatment option in patients with stable angina should have at
least one of the following goals:
- To improve prognosis
- To minimize or abolish symptoms
- To reduce the need for subsequent interventions.

Patients in whom catheterization reveals significant coronary artery
stenosis may be potential candidates for revascularization. In particular,
a patient is eligible for revascularization if:
- Optimal medical therapy is unsuccessful or not completely
  successful in controlling symptoms
- A large area of myocardium is at risk as identified by non-invasive tests

Table 8.1 Recommendations for coronary arteriography, for establishing a diagnosis (Table 8.1a) and for risk stratification (Table 8.1b) (adapted from ESC guidelines on the management of stable angina pectoris)

8.1a Recommendations for coronary arteriography for establishing a diagnosis in stable angina

Class I B	Severe stable angina (CCS ≥ 3), with a high pre-test probability of disease, particularly if not responders to medical treatment Survivors of cardiac arrest
Class I C	Serious ventricular arrhythmias Recurrency of angina in patients with previous PCI or coronary artery bypass grafting (CABG)
Class IIa C	Inconclusive or conflicting diagnosis on non-invasive testing if intermediate to high risk of coronary disease Previous PCI in a prognostically important site, at high risk of restenosis

8.1b Recommendations for coronary arteriography for risk stratification in stable angina

Class I B	High risk for adverse outcome on the basis of non-invasive testing independently of symptoms Severe stable angina (CCS ≥ 3), particularly if not responders to medical treatment Stable angina in patients who are being considered for major non-cardiac surgery, especially vascular, with intermediate or high risk on non-invasive testing
Class IIa C	Patients with an inconclusive or conflicting diagnosis on non-invasive testing Previous PCI in a prognostically important site, at high risk of restenosis

- The likelihood of success is high and the risks of morbidity and mortality are acceptable
- Patient's agreement, once he or she has been fully informed of risks and benefits of this kind of therapy.

The recommendations regarding myocardial revascularization as proposed by the ESC guidelines are listed in Table 8.2.

8.1.1. Indications for CABG

According to observational and randomized trial data comparing CABG with medical treatment, and to the current guidelines, larger benefits are observed with surgery in the presence of specific angiographic features, which are:

- Significant stenosis of the LMCA
- Significant proximal stenosis of all three major coronary arteries
- Significant stenosis of two major coronary arteries, including high-grade stenosis of the proximal LAD.

Table 8.2 Recommendations for myocardial revascularization (adapted and modified from ESC guidelines for treatment of chronic stable angina and ESC guidelines for PCI)

Recommendations for PCI When anatomy is suitable for PCI	
Indications	Classes of recommendation/ level of evidence
Angina CCS I–IV + single or multivessel CAD, non-diabetic	I A
Objective large ischaemia, even if minimal symptoms	I A; II B for prognosis
Chronic total occlusions (if symptoms + documented ischemia)	IIa C
High surgical risk/ left ventricular ejection fraction (LVEF) < 35%	IIa B
Angina CCS I–IV + multivessel CAD, diabetic	IIb C
Unprotected LMCA disease in absence of other options	IIb C
Recommendations for CABG When anatomy is suitable for surgery	
Indications	Classes of recommendation/ level of evidence
Angina CCS I–IV + LMCA disease or + 3 vessel disease + large ischemia or + 3 vessel disease + low LVEF or + 3-2 vessel disease with proximal LAD disease	I A
Angina CCS I–IV + multivessel CAD, diabetic	I B for symptoms; IIa B for prognosis

8.1.2 Indications for PCI

Modern stent design (flexible, low-profile, drug-eluting) and effective current adjuvant therapy allow to perform single or multivessel PCI with a high probability of success and with limited risk of complications. Thus, PCI may be indicated in all patients scheduled for revascularization, who are not indicated (see Section 8.1.1), not willing (they prefer PCI over surgery), or contraindicated to undergo coronary bypass surgery. This represents about 75% of all patients undergoing coronary revascularization.

8.1.3 PCI vs. medical therapy

A meta-analysis of randomized controlled trials found that PCI reduce angina compared with medical treatment, although the trials have not included enough patients for reliable estimates of the effect of PCI on MACE.

The recent COURAGE trial randomized 2287 patients to PCI with optimal medical therapy or to optimal medical therapy alone. No significant difference in outcomes were found. Long-term angina relief was only slightly more pronounced in the PCI group. The addition of PCI to optimal medical therapy reduced significantly the need of subsequent revascularization.

These data suggest that low-risk chronic stable patients may be managed with optimal medical therapy, whereas PCI is more effective in patients with larger extent of ischemic area, who are more symptomatic.

8.1.4 **PCI vs. CABG surgery**

Both PCI and CABG surgery improve the long-term outcomes of non-diabetic CAD patients to similar extent. The only difference is the higher number of repeated revascularization procedures after PCI. Additional data were published in 2009 by the SYNTAX trial.

8.2 **Adjunctive medications for PCI in stable CAD patients**

8.2.1 **Acetylsalicylic acid (ASA, aspirin)**

ASA should be given to all patients undergoing PCI, with the only exception of known allergy. If patients are not pre-treated, the recommended doses are 500 mg given orally more than 3 h prior to the intervention, or at least 300 mg intravenously at the time of the procedure. ASA should be given indefinitely after the PCI.

8.2.2 **Thienopyridines (e.g. clopidogrel)**

Thienopyridines use *after* stent implantation reduce the rate of acute and sub-acute stent thrombosis. All patients with bare metal stents (BMS) should use clopidogrel 75 mg/day during ≥4 weeks after PCI. All patients with DES should use clopidogrel during ≥12 months after PCI.

It is less clear, whether thienopyridines should be given *before* elective CAG (which may or may not be followed by ad-hoc PCI). The ESC guidelines recommend to pre-treat all patients undergoing elective CAG. The PRAGUE-8 trial showed that clopidogrel can be given safely in the catheterization laboratory between the two procedures (after CAG, before PCI).

8.2.3 **Unfractionated heparin (UFH)**

Its use is recommended during the standard PCI procedure, with a bolus dose of heparin of 100 units/kg, to maintain Activated Clotting Time between 250 and 350 s.

8.2.4 **Glycoprotein IIb/IIIa inhibitors**

PCI in stable CAD is quite a low-risk procedure as regard to thrombotic events. Therefore, GP IIb/IIIa receptor inhibitors are not recommended as part of the standard medication. They may otherwise be considered, in case of higher pre-procedural risk of ischemic complications, as unstable and complex lesions, or as bail-out additional drugs in case of no-reflow phenomenon, appearance of visible thrombus, or abrupt vessel closure.

8.2.5 **Direct thrombin inhibitors**

The use of a direct thrombin inhibitor such as bivalirudin to replace UFH or low molecular weight heparin (LMWH) is recommended only in patients with heparin-induced thrombocytopenia (HIT).

The classes of recommendation and levels of evidence for adjunctive therapy to PCI in chronic angina patients according to the current ESC guidelines are reported in Table 8.3.

Table 8.3 Recommendations for adjunctive therapy to PCI in chronic angina (adapted from ESC guidelines)

Class of drug	Dose–duration–situation	Class of recommendation
ASA	500 mg orally at least 3 h before PCI, or 300 mg i.v. directly before PCI	I B
	No more than 100 mg for chronic tx	
Thienopyridines (ticlopidine/clopidogrel)	Loading dose of 300 mg at least 6 h before PCI, ideally the day before, or 600 mg 2 h before PCI	I A
	For 3 to 4 weeks in addition to ASA after BMS implantation	I C
	For 6 to 12 months after drug-eluting stents (DES)	I C
	For 12 months after vascular brachytherapy	I C
UFH	100 units/kg if alone (ACT 250 to 350 s)	
	or 50 to 60 units/kg if added to GP IIb/IIIa inhibitors (ACT 200 to 250 s)	
LMWH	Limited data as sole Tx during PCI. No clear advantage over UFH	
GP IIb/IIIa inhibitors	Complex lesions, threatening/actual vessel closure, visible thrombus, no/slow reflow	II a C
Direct thrombin inhibitors	Bivalirudin to replace UFH or LMWHs in patients with HIT	I C

8.3 **Assessment of PCI results**

Successful PCI in elective patients is defined as residual stenosis of <20% with TIMI 3 flow, and without any adverse clinical events.

8.4 **PCI complications**

The current PCI technical success rate is >90%, mortality rate <1%, Q-wave myocardial infarction <2%, and emergency CABG need <1%. Features associated with an increased risk of the procedure are advanced age, female gender, unstable angina, depressed ventricular function, left main coronary disease, multivessel involvement, vessel tortuosity, heavy calcifications, complex coronary plaque.

Several lesion classifications have been proposed to identify patients at high-risk of procedural complications (Table 8.4).

Several complications may be observed during PCI, and are described elsewhere:

- Coronary rupture
- Extensive coronary dissection
- Distal embolization and/or no-reflow phenomenon
- Side-branch occlusion
- Intraprocedural coronary thrombosis
- Periprocedural cardiac enzyme release
- Contrast-induced nephropathy
- Bleeding complications.

8.4.1 **Troponin elevation after PCI**

After a PCI procedure in elective patients, troponin release is relatively common, occurring mainly in saphenous vein graft interventions, multi-stent placement, side-branch occlusion, or distal embolization.

Although elevated troponin has recently been reported to be a risk factor, a significant prognostic value for higher mortality is only observed if creatine kinase-MB (CK-MB) is higher than five times the normal value.

8.5 **Specific subgroups**

8.5.1 **Diabetes and multivessel disease (MVD)**

Diabetic patients have similar indications for revascularization as non-diabetics, but usually they have a rapidly progressive disease with high rates of multivessel involvement and restenosis. Many subgroup analyses of randomized trials have shown a worse outcome with PCI as compared to CABG for diabetic patients with multivessel disease, and this result was also confirmed for patients with MVD and high risk characteristics.

Table 8.4 Classification of coronary lesions
ACC/AHA LESION CLASSIFICATION SYSTEM   **Characteristics of type A, B1, B2, and C lesions**
Type A lesions (high success, >85%; low risk)   Discrete (<10 mm length)   Concentric   Readily accessible   Non-angulated segment <45°   Smooth contour   Little or no calcification   Less than totally occlusive   Not ostial in location   No major branch involvement   Absence of thrombus
Type B1 lesions (moderate success, 60% to 85%; moderate risk)   Tubular (10 to 20 mm length)   Eccentric   Moderate tortuosity of proximal segment   Moderately angulated segment, 45° to 90°   Irregular contour   Moderate to heavy calcification   Ostial in location   Bifurcation lesions requiring double guide wires   Some thrombus present   Total occlusion <3 months old
Type B2 lesions (Ellis modification of AHA/ACC system)   Two or more 'B' characteristics
Type C lesions (low success, <60%; high risk)   Diffuse (>2 cm length)   Excessive tortuosity of proximal segment   Extremely angulated segments, >90°   Inability to protect major side branches   Degenerated vein grafts with friable lesions   Total occlusion >3 months old

8.5.2. Previous bypass surgery

Patients with previous CABG can undergo a redo intervention if anatomy is suitable. It is important to consider that the risk of a second surgery is three times greater than the initial surgery and that there is an additional risk of damaging the internal mammary artery graft if present.

PCI can be performed either in the vein graft, arterial graft, or in the native coronary artery beyond the graft.

8.5.3 **Left main CAD**

Elective stenting of unprotected left main should be considered if there are no alternative revascularization options, or in case of very high peri-operative risks.

Recent studies and a meta-analysis have demonstrated the early and mid-term results of PCI in patients with unprotected LMCA. DES appears to be safe and feasible in selected patients, and might be more effective in preventing major adverse cardiac events, as compared with BMS. However, considering the limitations in reliability and the risk of DES thrombosis, more data from randomized trials are still needed, particularly in comparison with surgery which is currently still the treatment of choice.

8.6 **DES, restenosis, stent thrombosis**

The immediate outcomes of elective PCI in chronic stable CAD are generally excellent (see above). The major limitation was the restenosis rate (see also Chapter 7). Angiographic restenosis (>50% DS) is found within 6 months in 15% to 20% of all PCI with BMS implantation. Clinical restenosis (i.e. symptom recurrence) is present in only one-third to one-half of these patients, that is 5% to 10% of all PCI with BMS. No systemically (orally or intravenously) used drug can modify this risk. Local anti-proliferative drug delivery via a new stent generation—drug eluting stents (DES) have been proven to be highly effective in decreasing the restenosis rates. The DES enthusiasm was somewhat 'cooled down' by several reports showing a small (0.5% per year) increase in the risk of stent thrombosis. Stent thrombosis after BMS usually occurs within the initial 4 weeks after PCI, whereas in patients treated by DES it may occur as late as 2 yrs after PCI. Thus, DES is indicated in patients with higher restenosis risk, while patients at higher risk for stent thrombosis should be treated by BMS.

Key reading

Biondi-Zoccai GG, Lotrionte M *et al.* A collaborative systematic review and meta-analysis on 1278 patients undergoing percutaneous drug-eluting stenting for unprotected left main coronary artery disease. *Am Heart J* 2008; **155**: 274–83.

Boden WE, O'Rourke RA, Teo KK *et al.* for the COURAGE Trial Research Group. Optimal medical therapy with or without PCI for stable coronary disease. *N Engl J Med* 2007; **356**: 1503–16.

Bucher HC, Hengstler P, Schindler C, Guyatt GH. Percutaneous transluminal coronary angioplasty versus medical treatment for non-acute coronary heart disease: meta-analysis of randomised controlled trials. *BMJ* 2000; **321**: 73–7.

Brooks MM, Frye RL, Genuth S et al. Bypass Angioplasty Revascularization Investigation 2 Diabetes (BARI 2D) Trial Investigators. Hypotheses, design, and methods for the Bypass Angioplasty Revascularization Investigation 2 Diabetes (BARI 2D) Trial. Am J Cardiol 2006; **97**(12A): 9G–19G.

De Felice F, Fiorilli R, Parma A et al. Clinical outcome of patients with chronic total occlusion treated with drug-eluting stents. Int J Cardiol 28 January 2008 [Epub ahead of print].

Emond M, Mock MB, Davis KB et al. Long-term survival of medically treated patients in the Coronary Artery Surgery Study (CASS) Registry. Circulation 1994; **90**: 2645–57.

Fox K, Garcia MA, Ardissino D et al. Task Force on the Management of Stable Angina Pectoris of the European Society of Cardiology; ESC Committee for Practice Guidelines (CPG). Guidelines on the management of stable angina pectoris: executive summary The Task Force on the Management of Stable Angina Pectoris of the European Society of Cardiology. Eur Heart J 2006; **27**: 1341–81.

Guidelines for percutaneous coronary interventions. The Task Force for Percutaneous Coronary Interventions of the European Society of Cardiology. Eur Heart J 2005; **26**: 804–47.

Kini AS, Lee P, Marmur JD, Agarwal A, Duffy ME, Kim MC, Sharma SK. Correlation of postpercutaneous coronary intervention creatine kinase-MB and troponin I elevation in predicting mid-term mortality. Am J Cardiol 2004; **93**: 18–23.

Krone RJ, Laskey WK, Johnson C et al. for the Registry Committee of the Society for Cardiac Angiography and Interventions. A simplified lesion classification for predicting success and complications of coronary angioplasty. Am J Cardiol 2000; **85**: 1179–84.

Krone RJ, Shaw RE, Klein LW et al. ACC-National Cardiovascular Data Registry Evaluation of the American College of Cardiology/American Heart Association and the Society for Coronary Angiography and Interventions lesion classification system in the current "stent era" of coronary interventions (from the ACC-National Cardiovascular Data Registry). Am J Cardiol 2003; **92**: 389–94.

Mandadi VR, DeVoe MC, Ambrose JA et al. Predictors of troponin elevation after percutaneous coronary intervention. Am J Cardiol 2004; **93**: 747–50.

Moreno R, Fernandez C, Alfonso F et al. Coronary stenting versus balloon angioplasty in small vessels a meta-analysis from 11 randomized studies. J Am Coll Cardiol 2004; **43**: 1964–72.

Ong AT, Serruys PW, Mohr FW et al. The SYNergy between percutaneous coronary intervention with TAXus and cardiac surgery (SYNTAX) study: design, rationale and run-in phase. Am Heart J 2006; **151**: 1194–204.

Silber S, Albertsson P, Avilés FF et al. Guidelines for percutaneous coronary intervention: the task Force for Percutaneous Coronary Interventions of the European Society of Cardiology. Eur Heart J 2005; **26**: 806–47

Widimsky P, Motovská Z, Simek S *et al.* on behalf of the PRAGUE-8 trial Investigators. Clopidogrel pre-treatment in stable angina: for all patients >6 h before elective coronary angiography or only for angiographically selected patients a few minutes before PCI? A randomized multicentre trial PRAGUE-8. *Eur Heart J*, 25 April 2008 [Epub ahead of print].

Yusuf S, Zucker D, Peduzzi P *et al.* Effect of coronary artery bypass graft surgery on survival: overview of 10-year results from randomised trials by the Coronary Artery Bypass Graft Surgery Trialists Collaboration. *Lancet* 1994; **344**: 563–70.

Chapter 9

PCI for acute coronary syndromes (including STEMI)

Petr Widimsky

> ### Key points
>
> - Acute coronary syndromes represent the most important indication for percutaneous coronary intervention (PCI) due to the fact that only for this group of patients PCI is proved as life-saving therapy.
> - Technique is similar to elective PCI in stable patients.
> - The organization of the entire team and infrastructure plays a critical role.

9.1 Primary PCI for ongoing acute myocardial infarction with ST elevation

Figure 9.1 shows the recommended strategy for the initial treatment of acute coronary syndromes. Primary PCI was shown to be the most effective treatment of acute myocardial infarction. To achieve this high effectivity, certain organizational aspects should be strictly followed.

Pre-hospital care. Patients should be transferred directly 'first medical contact—cath-lab', bypassing the nearest non-PCI hospital and bypassing the emergency room (ER) or coronary care unit (CCU) in the PCI hospital. The drugs used in the pre-hospital care include aspirin, heparin, and clopidogrel.

Regional networks and transfer for primary PCI. Transfer for primary PCI decreased 30-day mortality from 8.9% (thrombolysis) to 7.0% (transfer for PCI), recurrent myocardial infarction from 6.7% to 1.8%, and stroke from 2.2% to 1.1% in five trials performed in four different countries.

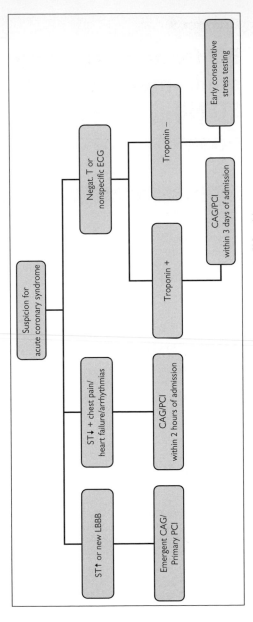

Figure 9.1 Acute coronary syndrome (ACS) initial decision-making algorithm. Modified from the ESC guidelines.

Table 9.1 Optimal vs. real-life time delays in primary PCI networks

Time intervals	Ideally	Real life
Pain–call	5 min	1–10 h
Call–arrival	<15 min	10–30 min
On-site examination including electrocardiogram (ECG)	<15 min	10–20 min
Transfer to nearest small hospital (first door)	Should not exist	10–45 min
Exam in small hospital (door-in–door-out)	Should not exist	20–60 min
Transfer to PCI centre (second door)	<60 min.	20–60 min
Exam in CCU or ER of PCI centre	Should not exist	20–30 min
Cath-lab (third) door–balloon inflation	<30 min	<30 min
Total ischemic time	<2 h	3–12 h

In **bold** are the intervals, where logistics has yet to be substantially improved.
In *italics* are those intervals where medical services usually operate very effectively.

Time delays. The ideal vs. real-life time delays are in Table 9.1. Proper co-ordination between all segments (emergency services–referral hospitals–ER/CCU in PCI hospitals–cath-labs), strict discipline of the entire team, and ongoing quality control focused on time delays are essential in achieving the highest standards of care.

Primary vs. facilitated vs. rescue vs. late PCI. Primary PCI is defined as emergent PCI performed for an ongoing acute myocardial infarction with ST-segment elevations (STEMI) usually within <12 h from symptom onset, without thrombolysis. The term 'facilitated PCI' is used for the planned combination of intravenous thrombolysis with subsequent (immediate) emergent PCI. Rescue PCI is PCI performed for ongoing myocardial infarction after unsuccessful thrombolysis (i.e. performed only in selected patients in whom thrombolysis clinically failed—and thus per definition is done with longer delay than facilitated PCI). Late PCI for myocardial infarction is done after >24 h from symptom onset. Primary PCI is the treatment of choice for STEMI today. Only for those regions, where primary PCI is not available, pre-hospital thrombolysis should be the second option (combined with immediate transfer to PCI centre).

Technique and material selection. Procedure begins by a diagnostic catheter imaging the non-infarct artery and then the guiding catheter is used for the infarct artery imaging and PCI (Figure 9.2). After CAG, the

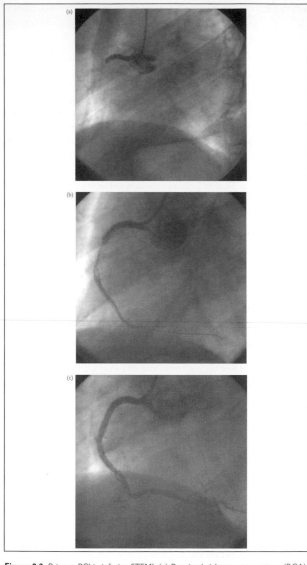

Figure 9.2 Primary PCI in inferior STEMI. (a) Proximal right coronary artery (RCA) occlusion. (b) Partial flow (TIMI-2) restored after guide wire passage through the occlusion, large intraluminal thrombus clearly visible. (c) Optimal PCI result with TIMI-3 flow after the implantation of 4.0/24 mm stent (Liberté®).

cardiologist must be absolutely certain about the culprit lesion before starting PCI. Intracoronary guide wire with soft tip is usually used, as most occlusions during the acute phase of STEMI are soft with fragile clots, which can be easily and safely crossed by a soft-tip guide wire. Direct stenting is advisable whenever the distal segment is sufficiently visualized after guide wire passage and when stent size can be precisely selected. Balloon predilatation is recommended in all other situations. Balloon should be first (before the first inflation) advanced distally and withdrawn back in its deflated state. This simple 'Dotter-like' manoeuver is useful for two reasons: (1) to ensure the guide wire position in the distal segment of the infarct artery (instead of a side branch or pericardium) and (2) to exclude the possibility that stenosis (to be dilated) is distal to the angiographic occlusion site (proximal thrombus apposition may lead to balloon inflation in the thrombus, but not in the most critical stenosis, resulting in no-reflow in some patients).

The use of other devices (thrombectomy, distal protection, etc.) in primary PCI is subject of ongoing debate. Their routine use cannot be recommended and they are not included in this book. Manual aspiration thrombectomy is increasingly used after the results of the TAPAS trial.

Multivessel PCI in the acute phase of myocardial infarction is discouraged by the ESC guidelines. It can be advocated only in the rare patient with two critical stenoses (occlusions), when the investigator is unable to distinguish which one is the culprit lesion. Stable contra-lateral lesion (even if high grade by diameter stenosis) should not be treated in the acute phase.

Coronary flow and myocardial perfusion. The goal of primary PCI in STEMI is to restore the coronary flow and myocardial perfusion. For practical purpose, the coronary flow is described in the simple TIMI-flow scale: TIMI-0 means no flow distal to the occlusion site; TIMI-1 is a slight contrast 'staining' in the short segment just behind the occlusion with no visible flow in the distal segments of the artery. TIMI-2 means delayed, but complete filling of the coronary artery, and TIMI-3 is normal flow. 'TIMI frame count' is a simple tool to quantify this more by counting the number of frames needed for the contrast to reach the distal segments of the coronary artery. Myocardial perfusion can be evaluated as a simple 'myocardial blush grade'.

Cardiogenic shock, pulmonary oedema. Primary PCI decreased 30-day mortality of STEMI patients, who present without any signs of heart failure to 0.5%–2%. The mortality of patients presenting in heart failure (Killip II–IV class) was also substantially decreased by the use of primary PCI, but still remains high: 40% to 50% for Killip IV (cardiogenic shock) patients and 20% to 30% for Killip III (pulmonary oedema patients). Especially frustrating are the outcomes of elderly (>75 yrs) STEMI patients in cardiogenic shock—their mortality is 70% to 75% despite primary PCI. Thus, the best therapy of cardiogenic shock is to prevent its development by the fast-track transfer of STEMI patients to cath-lab (before the shock will eventually develop). Most patients in Killip III–IV class have to be stabilized by intubation and artificial ventilation before the PCI procedure, some of them need intra-aortic balloon pump (IABP). When these measures are taken at the CCU with the goal to stabilize the patient before he (she) is taken to cath-lab, at least 30 min (sometimes over 1 h) time is lost. Thus, we always intubate the patients (and insert IABP when necessary) in the cath-lab simultaneously with the introduction of arterial sheath and first diagnostic catheter. We never introduce IABP before PCI—our aim is always to open the artery as fast as possible. Only when haemodynamic situation does not improve after PCI do we consider IABP use.

Temporary pacemaker insertion during primary PCI procedure is very rarely needed. Bradycardias (including complete heart block) usually resolve spontaneously and promptly after reperfusion. Thus, our strategy is always to do the first balloon inflation as fast as possible and postpone the decision about temporary pacemaker (and also about IABP) to few minutes after the infarct artery was opened.

STEMI caused by stent thrombosis. Stent thrombosis is a rare (~1%), but feared complication of stent placement. Unlike restenosis (which is a slow and usually benign process, resulting in repeat revascularization), stent thrombosis is an emergent event, resulting in death (mortality 18% to 45% in different reports) or left ventricular (LV) dysfunction. Acute and subacute stent thrombosis occurs with similar frequency after DES and BMS implantation and is usually caused by suboptimal stent deployment and/or ineffective thienopyridine therapy (clopidogrel resistance or interruption). Late stent thrombosis occurs almost exclusively after DES implantation and is the reason for long (at least 12 months) clopidogrel treatment in this setting. The treatment of stent thrombosis is emergent re-PCI (Figure 9.3).

9.2 PCI for non-ST elevation acute coronary syndromes

Patients with ongoing or recurrent chest pain and ST-segment depressions should be treated in the same way as STEMI patients: that is fast track to the cath-lab for CAG (Figure 9.4). Coronary bypass grafting can be a good option for these patients (~15%) when coronary anatomy is not suitable for PCI. PCI is preferred whenever the infarct artery can be easily defined and the lesion is amenable for PCI (~60% of patients) or when severe haemodynamic compromise does not allow enough time for cardiac surgery (Figures 9.5 and 9.6).

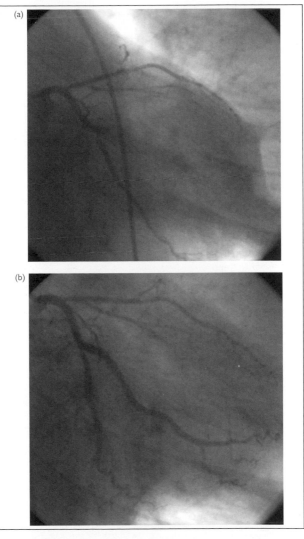

Figure 9.3 Acute inferolateral ST-depression myocardial infarction caused by the thrombosis of a 3.5/18 mm stent implanted 2 weeks ago to the proximal segment of the obtuse marginal artery. Caudal view. This patient deliberately stopped Plavix® after hospital discharge (4 days after the original PCI and 10 days before this event). (a) Proximal 100% OM occlusion. (b) Optimal result after dilatation with a 4.0/20 mm balloon (Maverick®) and full antithrombotic medication including heparin, Integrilin®, and Aspegic®.

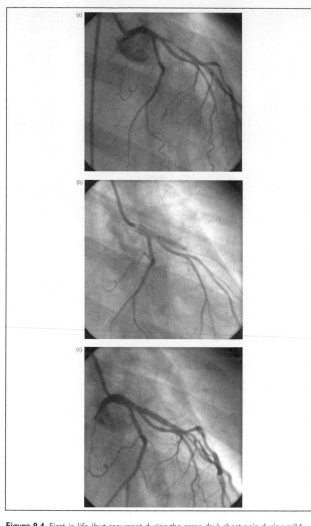

Figure 9.4 First-in-life (but recurrent during the same day) chest pain during mild exercise brought this young top manager to the hospital late afternoon. No ECG changes were found (ECG was done when he was without symptoms), he was admitted due to the high risk of coronary artery disease (family history, smoking, hypertension) with the diagnosis possible unstable angina. (a) Proximal 90% left anterior descending (LAD) stenosis with smooth margins. (b) Direct stenting of this lesion was easy. The contrast shot was used to control the position of the implanted stent with respect to the intermediate branch and left main. (c) Final result shows ideal slight oversizing (negative residual stenosis).

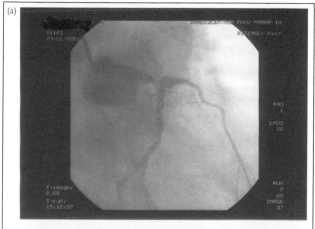

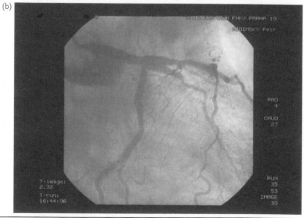

Figure 9.5 Critical (95%) LMCA stenosis and acute 100% ostial LAD occlusion in a patient with cardiogenic shock.(a) Only intermediate branch and LCX artery are visualized distally to the LMCA stenosis. Occluded LAD cannot be seen. It is of crucial importance to recognize this immediately (and not to misinterpret the intermediate branch as small LAD!). (b) Final result after emergency T-stenting. After double wire protection, balloon (2.5/20 mm Maverick®) predilatation LMCA to LAD was done, followed by 4.0/20 mm stent (TaxusLiberté®) implantation from LMCA to proximal LAD and finally MultilinkVision® 3.5/13 mm stent was implanted to the proximal segment of the intermediate branch. Not only LAD was opened successfully, but also the big diagonal branch is now visible and of course the LMCA stenosis was treated.

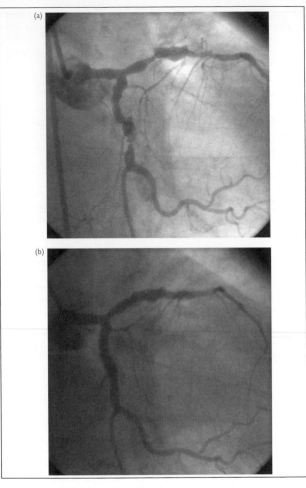

Figure 9.6 Acute ST-depression myocardial infarction complicated by pulmonary oedema in 75-yrs-old diabetic lady after old inferior Q-MI (with chronic total occlusion of the RCA). (a) The culprit (unstable) lesion is very likely the left circumflex: this stenosis shows typical characteristics of an acutely unstable lesion (critical, hazy, exulcerated, with intraluminal lucencies). The proximal LAD stenosis is also significant, but seems to be chronic stable lesion. This angiographic conclusion was supported by ECG changes predominantly on the lateral wall. This can serve as an example, that simple (semi)quantitative description of percent diameter stenosis is not sufficient: by contours, the LCX lesion can be assessed as 60% and the LAD as 80%, but from qualitative description of these lesions it is understandable that LCX is the culprit. (b) Final result after stent implantation to both lesions (Liberté® 4.0/12 mm in LAD and Multilink Vision® 4.0/18 mm in LCX).

Patients in less urgent situations (i.e. those with full relief after initial medical therapy) are usually treated within 3 days of admission in a way technically similar to elective PCI. The indications for coronary angiography (CAG) in non-STE ACS based on the ESC guidelines 2007 are the following:

- Urgent CAG (<2 h after admission) in refractory/recurrent angina with dynamic ST deviation, heart failure, arrhythmias, or haemodynamic instability
- Early CAG (<3 days after admission) in initially stabilized patients with intermediate to high-risk features
- No routine CAG in patients without intermediate to high-risk features, but non-invasive assessment of inducible ischaemia is advised.

9.3 Periprocedural medication in PCI for acute coronary syndromes

Antiplatelet agents. Three types of these agents are used: acetylsalicylic acid (aspirin, ASA), thienopyridines (clopidogrel, ticlodipine [not licensed in the UK], in near future maybe prasugrel) and GPIIb/IIIa inhibitors (abciximab, eptifibatide, tirofiban). ASA and clopidogrel are used in all patients, GP IIb/IIIa inhibitors for the high risk STEMI patients in some countries and for all STEMI patients in others.

Anticoagulant drugs are also used with each PCI procedure. Heparin (UFH) has largest experience and best cost effectivity. The initial bolus dose is 100 units/kg body weight (or 50 to 60 units/kg if GPIIb/IIIa inhibitors are used). Target ACT is 250 to 350 s or APTT 60 to 80 s. Patients, who received LMWH (e.g. enoxaparin) before entering to cath-lab, should continue the same LMWH during the procedure (cath-lab dose based on the previous dose time). Combining UFH and LMWH causes more bleeding. On the other hand, patients previously treated by fondaparinux should receive additional UFH during the PCI procedure. Bivalirudin is a new and potent anticoagulant drug, which was shown to be superior to the combination UFH + GPIIb/IIIa inhibitors. However, it was never tested in a large randomized trial against UFH alone. Patients on chronic oral anticoagulation (warfarin) present a special problem when they suffer an acute coronary syndrome. In the emergent setting (e.g. STEMI), the 5F sheath, lower UFH dose and no GPIIb/IIIa inhibitors should be used. Sheath can be safely removed when INR is <2.0. With high INR (>3.0) fresh frozen plasma or closure device should be used.

Thrombolytics have been largely replaced by primary PCI in the treatment of STEMI patients. They have only one place in this setting: as immediate pre-hospital reperfusion therapy in those areas, where primary PCI cannot be done within 2 h of the first medical contact. Patients treated by pre-hospital thrombolysis in such areas should be transferred to PCI centre (and not to the nearest hospital) for subsequent CAG. Thrombolytics should never be used in cath-lab for opening the artery after failed PCI (such strategy may cause fatal complications—e.g. cardiac tamponade).

Other drugs used in the cath-lab during PCI in ACS (sedatives, analgetics, atropine, catecholamines, nitrates, beta-blockers, calcium antagonists) are given in standard clinical indications. It is especially important to use atropine (dose 0.5 to 1.0 mg i.v., maximal total dose 2 mg) immediately in vagal reactions (hypotension + bradycardia): atropine can reverse such reaction promptly, while failure to use atropine may cause severe problems (profound hypotension, resuscitation, temporary pacemaker insertion, and so on).

9.4 **Normal CAG in patients referred as suspected acute coronary syndromes**

Approximately 2% to 3% of patients presenting to the cath-lab as acute STEMI have normal coronary angiography. Majority (1.5% to 2%) have other cardiovascular pathology (pulmonary embolism, acute myocarditis, acute pericarditis, cardiomyopathies, aortic dissection, stress-induced myocardial stunning, hypertension), very few (~0.5%) have a real acute coronary syndrome (caused by transient spasm and/or thrombus, disappearing before CAG). In the non-ST-elevation setting, normal CAG can be found in up to 10% of patients (usually troponin-negative patients without diagnostic ECG changes) and many of these patients have non-cardiac diseases.

9.5 **Complications of PCI in acute coronary syndromes**

Periprocedural mortality. In-hospital mortality (related to the disease, not to the procedure) of non-selected consecutive STEMI patients undergoing primary PCI is between 5% and 10%. It is increased with age >75 yrs, with Killip class >I and with low experience or poor organization of the PCI centre. Centres reporting mortality rates for primary PCI below 5% almost always do some patient selection (exclude very elderly patients, exclude terminal cardiogenic shock or post-resuscitation patients, etc.). In-hospital mortality of patients undergoing PCI for non-ST-elevation ACS is ~1%–2%.

Mechanical complications. Mechanical complications are caused by either inexperienced (or not fully concentrated) interventional cardiologist or by the risky anatomy of the patient (heavy calcifications, extreme vessel tortuosity, and so on). Which complications can be encountered during the primary PCI procedure?

The most feared is coronary rupture with subsequent haemopericardium and cardiac tamponade. This (usually fatal in the setting of STEMI) complication can be caused by inadverent balloon inflation in the vessel wall (i.e. guide wire was introduced into the wall and is not distally in the infarct vessel lumen) or in a significantly smaller branch (which is mistakenly considered to be the infarct artery—e.g. 3.5 mm balloon inflated in 1 mm septal branch or diagonal instead of intended 3.5 mm LAD). This is typical for inexperienced low volume operators. This complication is very difficult to recognize even at the autopsy: autopsy finding usually confirms large acute myocardial infarction (for which the primary PCI was planned) with haemopericardium (which is usually attributed by the pathologist to the ruptured LV free wall). Treatment is immediate balloon occlusion of the artery segment just proximally to the rupture, pericardiocentesis, and sometimes (when time and artery diameter allows) stent-graft or emergent surgery.

Other (very rare) complications may include aortic dissection by the guiding catheter, spiral coronary dissection by the guiding catheter, air embolism, thrombotic embolization from the guiding catheter, and so on.

Bleeding complications. These are much more frequent after PCI in acute coronary syndromes than after elective PCI in chronic stable coronary artery disease. The reason is mainly the higher dosage and combination use of antithrombotic drugs in the acute setting. Most severe bleeding complications occur in three situations:

- In elderly patients with low body weight (mostly such patients are females)
- After thrombolytics use (facilitated PCI, rescue PCI)
- GPIIb/IIIa inhibitors are combined with high dose of heparin.

Perforation of the great vessels is usually a typical complication of an inexperienced operator, it almost never happens to skilled experienced operators. Angiography, CT scan confirm these complications. Blood and volume replacement, correction of coagulation plasma factors as first step treatment could be in most cases successful.

Retroperitoneal haematomas are uncommon and are usually caused by puncture of the distal external iliac artery (too 'high'—proximal–arterial puncture). The use of large catheters (>6 F), longer procedure times and full-dose/multiple combination antithrombotic drugs use increase the risk of this complication. Patients with this complication become usually hypotensive or shocked, they have often no signs of haematoma or any other complication at the inguinal puncture site. CT scan confirms retroperitoneal haematoma.

Access site haematomas. In most cases, careful compression by an experienced member of staff and conservative management is sufficient, but rarely blood transfusion and surgical evacuation may be required. The occurrence of haematoma relates to several factors, including chosen puncture site, operator experience, device size, and use of anticoagulation.

Closure devices. Variety mechanical devices are now available to assist in haemostasis and puncture site closure (FemoStop®, Angioseal®, Perclose®, etc.). These closure devices may improve the patient comfort, they have not been shown to decrease significantly the complications rate.

Key reading

Andersen HR, Nielsen TT, Rasmussen K et al. A comparison of coronary angioplasty with fibrinolytic therapy in acute myocardial infarction. N Engl J Med 2003; **349**(8): 733–42.

ESC guidelines for percutaneous coronary interventions. *Eur Heart J* 2005; **26**: 804–47.

ESC guidelines for the diagnosis and treatment of non-ST segment elevation acute coronary syndromes. *Eur Heart J* 2007; **28**: 1598–660.

ESC guidelines on management of acute myocardial infarction in patients presenting with persistent ST-segment elevation. *Eur Heart J* 2008; **29**: 2909–45.

Grines CL et al. A randomized trial of transfer for primary angioplasty versus on-site thrombolysis in patients with high-risk myocardial infarction. The Air Primary Angioplasty in Myocardial Infarction Study. *J Am Coll Cardiol* 2002; **39**: 1713–19.

Keeley EC, Boura JA, Grines CL. Primary angioplasty versus intravenous thrombolytic therapy for acute myocardial infarction: a quantitative review of 23 randomised trials. *Lancet* 2003; **361**: 13–20.

Vermeer F, Oude Ophuis AJ, vd Berg EJ et al. Prospective randomized comparison between thrombolysis, rescue PTCA, and primary PTCA in patients with extensive myocardial infarction admitted to a hospital without PTCA facilities: a safety and feasibility study. *Heart* 1999; **82**: 426–31.

Widimský P, Budesinsky T, Vorac D et al. 'PRAGUE' Study Group Investigators. Long distance transport for primary angioplasty vs immediate thrombolysis in acute myocardial infarction. Final results of the randomized national multicentre trial—PRAGUE-2. *Eur Heart J* 2003; **24**(1): 94–104.

Widimský P, Groch L, Želízko M, Aschermann M, Bednář F, Suryapranata H. Multicenter randomized trial comparing transport to primary angioplasty vs. immediate thrombolysis vs. combined strategy for patients with acute myocardial infarction presenting to a community hospital without a catheterization laboratory. The PRAGUE Study. *Eur Heart J* 2000; **21**: 823–31.

Chapter 10

Percutaneous valvular interventions

Dominique Himbert, Gregory Ducrocq,
Alec Vahanian

Key points

- The technique of percutaneous valve dilatation has
  proven efficacy in the treatment of mitral stenosis as a
  substitute for surgical commissurotomy and as a
  complement to valve replacement.
- Aortic valvuloplasty probably has a very limited role in
  isolation but may find new applications as the first step
  in the performance of percutaneous aortic valve
  replacement.
- Transcatheter aortic valve implantation is a new and
  promising technique for patients with aortic stenosis and
  unacceptable risk for surgery. It is still in its infancy and
  careful evaluation is needed before defining the precise
  role of the technique.

10.1 Percutaneous mitral commissurotomy (PMC)

Performance of PMC should be restricted to centres whose experience with transseptal catheterization has been positive and who have
been able to carry out an adequate number of procedures and thus
improve their technical performance and ability to select patients.

10.1.1 Indications and contraindications

10.1.1.1 Indications for PMC

The decision to perform valvuloplasty must be based on both clinical
and anatomic variables. For symptomatic patients, the indication for
PMC is summarized in Figure 10.1. Truly asymptomatic patients,
however, are not usually candidates for the procedure because of
the small but definite risk inherent in the technique. For patients in
this latter group, PMC may be considered in selected cases: patients

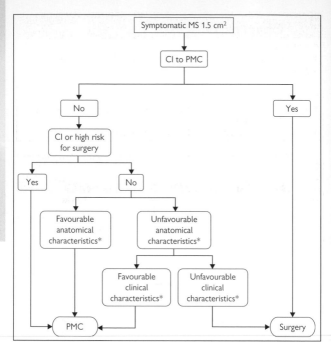

Figure 10.1 Management of severe symptomatic mitral stenosis ≤1.5 cm².
*Favourable characteristics for percutaneous mitral commissurotomy can be defined by the absence of several of the following unfavourable characteristics: clinical characteristics: old age, history of commissurotomy, NYHA class IV, atrial fibrillation, severe pulmonary hypertension; anatomic characteristics: echo score >8, Cormier score 3 (Calcification of mitral valve of any extent, as assessed by fluoroscopy), very small mitral valve area, severe tricuspid regurgitation.

at high risk of thromboembolism; previous history of embolism; or heavy spontaneous contrast in the left atrium (LA)—recurrent atrial arrhythmias—Guidelines also recommend PMC at this stage when systolic pulmonary pressures is higher than 50 mmHg at rest. Finally, PMC can be considered for patients requiring major extra cardiac surgery or to allow for pregnancy.

10.1.1.2 *Contraindications*

Before performance of PMC clinical and echocardiographic assessment are needed to eliminate contraindications (Table 10.1) and evaluate prognosis. Echocardiography allows the classification of patients into anatomic groups. Most investigators use the Wilkins score for categorization (Table 10.2), whereas others use a more general assessment of valve anatomy (Table 10.3).

Table 10.1 Contraindications to percutaneous mitral commissurotomy

- Mitral valve area > 1.5 cm²
- Left atrial thrombus
- More than mild mitral regurgitation
- Severe- or bicommissural calcification
- Absence of commissural fusion
- Severe concomitant aortic valve disease, or severe combined tricuspid stenosis and regurgitation
- Concomitant coronary artery disease requiring bypass surgery

Table 10.2 Anatomic scores predicting outcome after percutaneous mitral commissurotomy: Wilkins' mitral valve morphology score

Grade	Mobility	Subvalvular thickening	Thickening
1	Highly mobile valve with only leaflet tips restricted	Minimal thickening just below the mitral leaflets	Leaflets near normal in thickness (4–5 mm)
2	Leaflet mid and base portions have normal mobility	Thickening of chordal structures extending to one third of the chordal length	Midleaflets normal, considerable thickening of margins (5–8 mm)
3	Valve continues to move forward in diastole, mainly from the base	Thickening extended to distal third of the chords	Thickening extending through the entire leaflet (5–8 mm)

Adapted from Wilkins GT, Weyman AE, Abascal VM, Block PC, Palacios IF. Percutaneous balloon dilatation of the mitral valve: an analysis of echocardiographic variables related to outcome and the mechanism of dilatation. *Br Heart J* 1988; **60**: 299–308.

Table 10.3 Anatomic scores predicting outcome after percutaneous mitral commissurotomy: Cormier's grading of mitral valve anatomy

Echocardiographic group	Mitral valve anatomy
Group 1	Pliable non-calcified anterior mitral leaflet and mild subvalvular disease (i.e. thin chordae ≥10 mm long)
Group 2	Pliable non-calcified anterior mitral leaflet and severe subvalvular disease (i.e. thickened chordae <10 mm long)
Group 3	Calcification of mitral valve of any extent, as assessed by fluoroscopy, whatever the state of subvalvular apparatus

Adapted from Iung B, Cormier B, Ducimetiere P, Porte JM, Nallet O, Michel PL, Acar J, Vahanian A. Immediate results of percutaneous mitral commissurotomy. A predictive model on a series of 1514 patients. *Circulation* 1996; **94**: 2124–30.

10.1.2 **Technique**

10.1.2.1 *Transseptal catheterization*

Transseptal catheterization, which allows access to the LA, is the first step in the procedure and one of the most crucial. The *Inoue technique* is now almost exclusively used. A specific guide wire with a J-shaped distal part is introduced into the LA via a transseptal catheter, which is then withdrawn. Subsequently, a dilator (14Fr) is passed along the guide wire to dilate both the entry site and the interatrial septum. Finally, the Inoue balloon is inserted on the guide wire (Figure 10.2). Balloon size should be chosen according to patient height. When the balloon is placed in the LA the guide wire is withdrawn and replaced by a stylet, which helps to direct the balloon towards the mitral valve. Intravenous heparin is given (3000 units). It is recommended to use a stepwise dilatation technique under echocardiographic guidance.

10.1.2.2. *Echocardiographic monitoring*

Echocardiographic monitoring provides essential information on the efficacy of the procedure and also enables early detection of complications. The following criteria have been proposed for the desired end point of the procedure: (a) mitral valve area greater than 1 cm^2 per square meter of body surface area, (b) complete opening of at

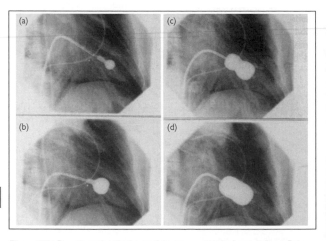

Figure 10.2 Percutaneous mitral commissurotomy using the Inoue balloon. Rao 30° view. Sequence of inflation of the Inoue balloon. (a) The distal tip of the balloon is inflated and allows crossing of the mitral valve. (b) The distal part of the balloon is further inflated and pulled backward. (c) Further inflation is performed allowing for inflation of the proximal part of the balloon. The balloon is located at the level of the mitral valve. The waist in the middle of the balloon is due to mitral stenosis. (d) The balloon is fully inflated and the waist disappears.

least one commissure, or (c) appearance or increment of regurgitation greater than 1/4 classification. When the result is judged to be final the stylet is withdrawn and replaced by the guide wire and the balloon is then withdrawn. Echocardiography using the transoesophageal approach, or more recently intracardiac probes, may facilitate the performance of the procedure, especially the transseptal puncture in difficult cases or when the operator is less experienced. For the final assessment, calculation of the valve area may be done using planimetry; and the degree of regurgitation may be established by angiography or Doppler colour flow imaging. The most sensitive method for the assessment of iatrogenic interatrial shunting is Doppler colour flow imaging.

10.1.3 Immediate results

PMC usually provides an increase of over 100% in valve area. Overall good immediate results (final valve area >1.5 cm² without mitral regurgitation >2/4) are observed in >80% of cases. The failure rate is 1% to 17%, procedural mortality 0% to 3%, haemopericardium 0.5% to 12%, embolism 0.5% to 5% of cases. The frequency of severe mitral regurgitation (requiring surgery) ranges from 2% to 12% (urgent surgery in only 1%). The iatrogenic interatrial shunts are usually small and without clinical consequences.

10.1.4 Long-term results

Late outcome after PMC differs according to the quality of the immediate results. Unsatisfactory immediate result usually means elective valve surgery. Successful immediate result remains stable in most patients, the risk of restenosis is 2% to 40% (occurring mostly within 3 to 5 yrs).

10.2 Percutaneous aortic valvuloplasty (PAV)

10.2.1 Indications for PAV

Aortic valve replacement is the standard treatment for symptomatic aortic stenosis. Valvuloplasty can be considered only in the following circumstances:

- Critically ill patients with cardiogenic shock with multivisceral failure. Good mid-term results have been obtained in limited series if surgical intervention was possible secondarily. For this group of patients, valvuloplasty can be considered a bridge to surgery, permitting the secondary operation with less risk
- Severe, poorly tolerated aortic stenosis requiring significant emergency non-cardiac surgery
- More rarely, in patients who have an absolute, but not life-threatening, short-term contraindication to surgery and have significant functional disability.

10.2.2 **Technique**

After retrograde crossing of the aortic valve, an extra-stiff Amplatz 0.035-inch, 270-cm guide wire is used to replace the crossing cathe-ter. Before use, a large, pigtail-shaped curve is formed at the distal end of the wire.

For valvuloplasty one may use the Z-Med II balloon catheter (12 to 14Fr sheath), or the lower-profile Cristal balloons (10Fr sheath). The diagnostic catheter is removed from the LV over the extra-stiff wire while the looped flexible segment of the wire is carefully maintained in the LV cavity. The 8Fr sheath is replaced by the 10Fr sheath over the extra-stiff wire. The balloon is advanced up to the descending aorta and carefully purged, then advanced across the aortic valve.

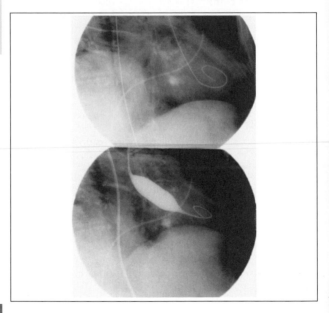

Figure 10.3 PAV. RAO 30° view. After crossing the aortic valve (upper panel) and introducing a stiff guide wire with a J tip in the LV, the balloon is inflated across the valve (lower panel).

Rapid (200 to 220/min) ventricular pacing can be used to arrest the forceful contractions of the heart thereby allowing the operator to stabilize the balloon in the optimal position (Figure 10.3). It is turned on, and balloon inflation is started quickly and with enough pressure to rapidly inflate the balloon as soon as the blood pressure falls. Balloon deflation is quickly performed, the pacer is turned off, and the balloon is withdrawn from the valve. Rapid balloon deflation and restoration of blood flow is important to minimize the duration of hypotension and hypoperfusion in these haemodynamically compromised patients. The residual gradient is then obtained. At this time, aortic angiography may be performed to determine the presence and/or severity of aortic regurgitation.

Manual compression is used for haemostasis at the venous entry site. With the use of the 14Fr sheath the previously placed Perclose sutures are used to close the arterial puncture. Now, the femoral artery access site is closed using an 8Fr Angioseal device whenever the 10Fr sheath has been used. If a technical failure occurs, a pneumatic pressure device is used. If the case is uncomplicated, the patient is usually discharged within 2 days.

10.2.3 Immediate results

Overall, PAV reduces tight stenosis to moderate stenosis. Hospital mortality is 3.5% to 13.5% and 20% to 25% of patients have at least one serious complication within the first 24 h (mostly vascular at the puncture site). Ventricular perforations could lead to tamponade. Acute aortic incompetence or embolic complications are rare.

10.2.4 Long-term results

Despite a relatively modest improvement in valve function, a degree of functional improvement is commonly noted during the first weeks. The benefit, however, disappears after a few months. Overall, the opinion is now that PAV alone does not change the natural course of the disease even after repeated procedures.

10.3 Transcatheter aortic valve implantation (TAVI)

Six years after the first in man by A. Cribier, TAVI for the treatment of aortic stenosis currently represents a dynamic field of research and development. Two devices have been CE marked and are commercialized. However, data are still reported mostly in oral communications and only few in peer-reviewed journals, which should be taken into account in their analysis.

At the present stage TAVI should be performed only in high volume centres, which have both cardiology and cardiac surgery departments, with expertise in structural heart disease intervention and high-risk valvular surgery. The procedure requires the close co-operation of a team of specialists in valve disease including clinical cardiologists, echocardiographists, interventional cardiologists, cardiac surgeons, and anaesthesiologists.

10.3.1 **Indications for TAVI**

Selection of candidates for TAVI should involve multi-disciplinary consultation between cardiologists, surgeons, imaging specialists, anaesthesiologists, and so on. TAVI is indicated in severely sympto-matic patients with calcified severe aortic stenosis, with extreme surgical risk (expected mortality >20% with the logistic EuroScore and >10% with STS score) or have contraindications to surgery.

The following steps should be taken initially to assess the feasibility of TAVI: Coronary angiography, angiography (or CT) of the pelvic arteries and aorta, TTE and TEE to assess the indication and any present contraindications.

10.3.2 **Contraindications for TAVI**

Contraindications for TAVI are: aortic annulus <18 mm or >25 mm for balloon expandable and <20 or >27 for self-expandable devices; bicuspid valves; presence of asymmetric heavy valvular calcification, which may compress the coronary arteries during TAVI; presence of bulky atherosclerosis of the ascending aorta; aortic root dimension >45 mm at the aorto-tubular junction for self-expandable prostheses; and presence of apical LV thrombus. Contraindications to femoral access are:

- At the iliac arteries: Severe calcification, tortuosity, small diameter (<6 to 9 mm according to the device used), and previous aorto-femoral bypass.
- At the aorta: Severe angulation, severe atheroma of the arch, coarctation, and aneurysm of the abdominal aorta with protruding mural thrombus.

10.3.3 **Technique**

The Edwards-Sapien valve is a balloon-expandable stent with peri-cardial cusps available in 23 and 26 mm sizes (22 to 24Fr sheaths). The CoreValve Revalving System is a self-expanding, valved stent with porcine cusps available in 26 and 29 mm sizes (18Fr sheath). TAVI is currently carried out using two different approaches (retro-grade transfemoral and antegrade transapical). Here we shall describe the transfemoral approach only.

The procedure is performed under general anaesthesia, although sedation and analgesia may suffice for the transfemoral approach. Peri-procedural transoesophageal echocardiography monitoring is desirable to correctly position the valve as well as to detect compli-cations. Close attention should be paid to the vascular access.

The common femoral artery can be either prepared surgically or approached percutaneously. Echographically guided femoral access could be useful. Manipulation of the introductory sheaths should be careful and fluoroscopically guided. Depending on the size of the device, closure of the vascular access can be effected surgically or using a percutaneous closure device.

After crossing the aortic valve, valvuloplasty is performed to predilate the native valve and serves as a rehearsal for TAVI. Simultaneous rapid pacing decreases cardiac output, stabilizing the balloon during inflation. The position of the prosthesis at the aortic valve can be assessed using fluoroscopy to assess the level of valve calcification, aortography, and/or echocardiography (transoesophageal). When positioning is considered correct, the prosthesis is released. Rapid pacing is used at this stage in balloon expandable, but not in self-expanding devices (Figure 10.4). Immediately after TAVI, aortography and, whenever available, transoesophageal echocardiography are performed to assess the location and degree of aortic regurgitation, and the patency of the coronary arteries. The haemodynamic results are assessed using pressure recordings and/or echocardiography. After the procedure, the patients should stay in intensive care for at least 24 h and be closely monitored for several days especially as regards haemodynamics, vascular access, rhythm disturbances (especially late atrioventricular block), and renal function.

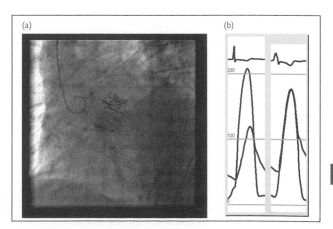

Figure 10.4 Transcatheter aortic valve implantation. (a) LAO 40° view. The aortic stented valve is positioned at the level of the aortic valve. (b) Pressure recording before (left) and after (right) TAVI.

10.3.4 **Results**

Procedural success is closely linked to experience, and is >90% in experienced centres. Valve function is good with a final valve area ranging from 1.5 to 1.8 cm^2. Mortality at 30 days is 5% to 18%, myocardial infarction occurs in 2% to 11% (coronary obstruction <1%), prosthesis embolization in 1%, stroke 3% to 9%. Mild to moderate aortic regurgitation (paravalvular) is observed in 50% of cases (severe aortic regurgitation in 5%). Vascular complications (10% to 15%) remain a significant cause of mortality and morbidity. Atrioventricular block occurs in 4% to 8%, necessitating pacemaker implantation in up to 24% with self-expandable devices.

Long-term results up to 2 yrs are reported in a limited number of patients. They show a survival rate of 70% to 80% with a significant improvement in clinical condition in most cases. The majority of late deaths are due to co-morbidities.

Serial echocardiographic studies have consistently shown good prosthetic valve function with no structural deterioration of valve tissue.

There are currently no direct comparative studies available of the two devices.

10.4 **Percutaneous mitral valve repair**

The new techniques of percutaneous mitral valve repair are at an early stage as they are still in evaluation and none are available outside of trials. The preliminary results, which currently relate to less than 300 patients treated worldwide, show us that these techniques are feasible and may result in an improvement in valve function. However, any further conclusions are speculative, and, thus, are out of the scope of this book.

Key reading

Cribier A, Letac B. Percutaneous balloon aortic valvuloplasty in adults with calcific aortic stenosis. Curr Opin Cardiol 1991; 6: 212–8.

Iung B, Baron G, Butchart EG et al. A prospective survey of patients with valvular heart disease in Europe: The Euro Heart Survey on Valvular Heart Disease. Eur Heart J 2003; 24: 1231–43.

Iung B, Cormier B, Ducimetiere P et al. Immediate results of percutaneous mitral commissurotomy. A predictive model on a series of 1514 patients. Circulation 1996; 94: 2124–30.

Iung B, Garbarz E, Michaud P et al. Late results of percutaneous mitral commissurotomy in a series of 1024 patients. Analysis of late clinical deterioration: frequency, anatomic findings, and predictive factors. Circulation 1999; 99: 3272–8.

Vahanian A, Alfieri O, Al-Attar N et al.; European Association of Cardio-Thoracic Surgery; European Society of Cardiology; European Association of Percutaneous Cardiovascular Interventions. Transcatheter valve implantation for patients with aortic stenosis: a position statement from the European Association of Cardio-Thoracic Surgery (EACTS) and the European Society of Cardiology (ESC), in collaboration with the European Association of Percutaneous Cardiovascular Interventions (EAPCI). Eur Heart J 2008; 29: 1463–70.

Vahanian A, Baumgartner H, Bax J et al.; Task Force on the Management of Valvular Hearth Disease of the European Society of Cardiology; ESC Committee for Practice Guidelines. Guidelines on the management of valvular heart disease: The Task Force on the Management of Valvular Heart Disease of the European Society of Cardiology. Eur Heart J 2007; 28: 230-68.

Vahanian A, Palacios IF. Percutaneous approaches to valvular disease. Circulation 2004; 109: 1572–9.

Webb JG, Pasupati S, Humphries K et al. Percutaneous transarterial aortic valve replacement in selected high-risk patients with aortic stenosis. Circulation 2007; 116: 755–63.

Chapter 11

Percutaneous interventions for congenital heart disease in adults

Jozef Mašura

Key points

- Percutaneous closure of congenital shunts (atrial septal defect (ASD) secundum type, foramen ovale patents, ventricular septal defect (VSD), and patent ductus arteriosus (PDA)) is feasible using modern implantable devices (e.g. Amplatzer occluders).
- Short-term results are excellent, long-term data comparing the outcomes with surgical treatment are not yet available.

11.1 ASD (ostium secundum) closure

Surgical closure of ostium secundum ASD is safe and effective with negligible mortality, but the morbidity associated with sternotomy/ thoracotomy, cardiopulmonary bypass, and potential for post-operative complications cannot be avoided. The studies of King and Mills (1974) began the way for the future development of transcatheter ASD device occlusion therapy. Several devices have been tested since that time. In 1997, a new self-expanding Nitinol prosthesis was developed and it consists of two self-expandable round disks connected to each other with a 4-mm wide waist and is commonly referred to as the Amplatzer septal occluder (ASO). Another device with attaching microsprings between the two umbrellas was named StarFlex. The final device of the decade was the Helex. It consists of a single Nitinol wire with a sleeve-like expanded polytetrafluoro-ethylene membrane attached to it. The wire is preshaped to form two disks that can be delivered transvenously. The currently utilized ASD occluding double-disk patch like devices have some limitations. The major disadvantages are the requirement of sufficient atrial septal rims, the need for the device size to be 1.5 to 2.0 times the

123

stretched ASD diameter, and complications related to wire components. Basically two types of devices are available: the patch-like devices and self-centric devices.

Transcatheter closure of ASD is an increasingly widespread alternative to surgical closure. The ASO is the most frequently used device for transcatheter closure of ASD (Figure 11.1). Short- and even long-term results of percutaneous closure of ASD using ASO are promising. Long-term data after ASO implantation are encouraging although some erosion of the surrounding structures with pericardial tamponade after implantation has been described.

11.1.1. **Implantation technique**

ASO implantation is performed via femoral vein and TEE monitoring is important. ASO is introduced via a long specific sheath through the defect to the left atrium, left disc is opened, positioned towards the left side of atrial septum. Then the right disk is opened and position is controlled. The atrial septum should be located between the two discs. For large ASD with deficient aortic rims, the left upper pulmonary

Figure 11.1 Implantation technique of ASO left disc with new AGA sheath. See the orientation of the septum and left disc in left anterior oblique (LAO) projection

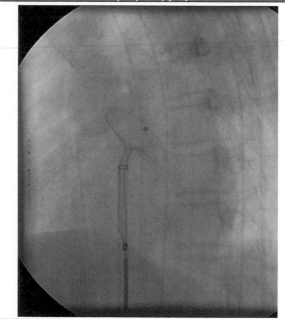

vein technique works well. In patients with deficient posterior rim the left atrial roof technique works quite well. There are other techniques described in the literature to avoid protrusion of the aortic edge of the device. These techniques, however, require an additional venous access, dilator tips, and balloons to keep the anterior edge from protruding into the right atrium. The description of these techniques is beyond the scope of this book.

11.2 Patent foramen ovale (PFO) closure

The foramen ovale is an opening in the septum secundum located inferoposteriorly and somewhat offset from the more superior and forward position of the ostium secundum. Together, the foramen ovale and ostium secundum form a one-way channel with the septum primum serving as a flap-valve, allowing the physiologic right-to-left shunting during intrauterine development. Autopsy series revealed that a PFO persists in 20% to 34% of the adults.

Recent studies indicate that paradoxical embolism through a PFO may be responsible for unexplained cerebrovascular accidents (CVAs) and transient ischaemic attacks (TIAs) in young adults. Long-term anticoagulation, surgical closure, and more recently, transcatheter occlusion of the PFO are available treatment options at the present time. Recently, the PFO was identified as an independent risk factor for mortality and a complicated in-hospital course in patients with major pulmonary embolism. The combination of PFO with stroke of undetermined cause (commonly referred to as cryptogenic) pertains to up to 40% of young stroke patients and has attracted much attention. The mechanism for right-to-left shunting via PFO in patients with paradoxical embolism, right ventricular infarction, or severe pulmonary disease is related to transient (phase after Valsalva manoeuver—for example, during coughing or defecation) or permanent pressure gradient (decreased right ventricular compliance following right ventricular infarction or increased pulmonary artery pressure in case of severe pulmonary disease).

11.2.1 Technique

The common construction principle of most devices consists of a double-umbrella design of various sizes closing the PFO by passive counter-tension against the atrial septal wall. The following description of the implantation procedure is limited to the steps common to most devices. The procedure is performed by transfemoral venous access under local anaesthesia. In contrast to percutaneous ASD closure, transesophageal monitoring is not routinely employed during device implantation. Similarly, measurements of the balloon-stretched diameter are optional, since they only rarely aid in device and size selection. Following administration of 5000 units systemic heparin, the PFO is crossed with a 6F (1F = 0.3 mm) multi-purpose catheter under fluoroscopic guidance in the anteroposterior (AP) view. This catheter is exchanged with a device-specific transseptal sheath measuring 8 to 12F. Air in the delivery system must be avoided by specific measures.

The constrained device is then introduced into the transseptal sheath and advanced to the tip of the catheter. First, the left atrial disk of the double umbrella is deployed and gently pulled back against the atrial septum. This and the following manoeuvers are best performed under fluoroscopic guidance in a LAO projection with some cranial angulation. To deploy the right atrial disk, tension is maintained on the delivery system, while the delivery sheath is further withdrawn. After a further Valsalva manoeuvre to produce back bleeding out of the sheath, a right atrial contrast angiography by a hand injection through the side arm of the delivery sheath serves to delineate the atrium septum. Upon verification of a correct position, the device is released from the delivery system. The transseptal sheath is used for a final contrast medium injection into right atrium. The contrast is followed to also delineate the left atrial contour and disk placement.

Percutaneous transseptal PFO closure is feasible. The question remains about its indications. The diagnosis of paradoxical embolism is usually difficult, the risk for stroke recurrence is poorly defined, and the long-term outcome of percutaneous PFO closure as compared with medical treatment and surgical PFO closure is unknown. Some concerns remain and include thrombus formation on the device surface, embolization of the device, late infections, and arrhythmias.

11.3 **PDA closure**

Operation, even for a small ductus in the adult, carries certain risk because the ductal wall may be calcified and can tear during ligation. In the present time the treatment of choice is closure of PDA with the use of intravascular closure devices and Amplatzer Ductal Occluder is the most commonly used (Figure 11.2). The procedure is safe with excellent results even in patients with borderline indication.

Percutaneous closure is an established method of treatment for the majority of patients with PDA. Currently, coils are the most widely used occluders for closure of small-sized PDA. For closure of moderate- and large-sized PDA, Amplatzer duct occluders are most often used. Immediate-, short-, and intermediate-term results of transcatheter PDA closure using ADO are excellent.

The selection of patients suitable for transcatheter closure using ADO was based solely on the measurement of the minimal PDA diameter on aortogram. Amplatzer duct occluders were selected for closure of PDA with a minimal diameter ≥2 mm. Coils are selected for closure of PDA with a minimal diameter <2 mm.

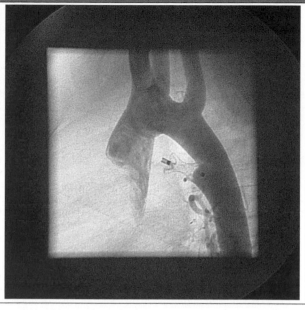

**Figure 11.2 Complete closure of PDA with ADO device.
Lateral view**

11.4 **VSD closure**

Morphological variation plays an important role during the device
selection. The incidence of residual shunt is up to 16%. During intermediate follow-up (3 to 24 months), the best results were found in
patients with a single hole defect without aneurysm. There are few
long-term data to establish the definite role of Amplatzer ventricular
septal occluder (Figures 11.3–11.5) in the treatment of *congenital
VSD* (compared with surgery).

Amplatz occluders (ventricular and also atrial type) have been
tested also in *post-infarction ventricular septal rupture*. The procedure
is feasible; however, the mortality of this feared MI complication
remains very high despite technically successful procedure.

Figure 11.3 Left ventricular angiogram after long sheath placement

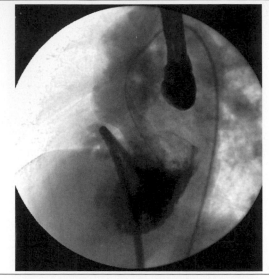

Figure 11.4 Implantation of Amplatzer VSD occluder in patients with aneurysm formation

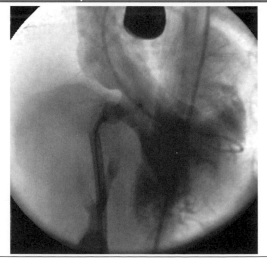

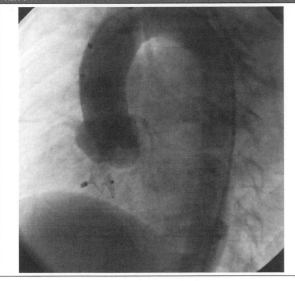

Figure 11.5 Final position of occluder just below the aortic valve

Key reading

Amin Z, Hijazi ZM, Bass JL, Cheatham JP, Hellenbrand WE, Kleinman CS. Erosion of Amplatzer septal occluder device after closure of secundum atrial septal defects: review of registry of complications and recommendations to minimize future risk. Catheter Cardiovasc Interv 2004; 63(4): 496–502.

Arora R, Trehan V, Kumar A, Kalra GS, Nigam M. Trancatheter closure of congenital ventricular septal defects experience with various devices. J Interv Cardiol 2003; 16(1): 83–91.

Butera G, Carminati M, Chessa M et al. Transcatheter closure of perimembranous ventricular septal defects: early and long-term results. J Am Coll Cardiol 2007; 50(12): 1189–95. Epub 2007 September 4.

Hijazi ZM, Hakim F, Haweleh AA et al. Catheter closure of perimembranous ventricular septal defects using the new Amplatzer membranous VSD occluder: initial clinical experience. Cathet Cardiovasc Interv 2002; 56: 508–15.

King TD, Mills NL. Nonoperative closure of atrial septal defects. Surgery 1974; 75(3): 383–8.

Masura J, Gao W, Gavora P et al. Percutaneous closure of perimembranous ventricular septal defects with the eccentric Amplatzer device: multicenter follow-up study. Pediatr Cardiol 2005; 26(3): 216–9.

Masura J, Gavora P, Formanek A, Hijazi ZM. Transcatheter closure of secundum atrial septal defects using the new self-centering amplatzer septal occluder: initial human experience. Cathet Cardiovasc Diagn 1997; 42(4): 388–93.

Masura J, Gavora P, Podnar T. Long-term outcome of transcatheter secundum-type atrial septal defect closure using Amplatzer septal occluders. J Am Coll Cardiol 2005; 45(4): 505–7.

Masura J, Tittel P, Gavora P, Podnar T. Long-term outcome of transcatheter patent ductus arteriosus closure using Amplatzer duct occluders. Am Heart J 2006; 151(3): 755.e7–755.e10.

Masura J, Walsh KP, Thanopoulous B *et al.* Catheter closure of moderate-to large-sized patent ductus arteriosus using the new Amplatzer duct occluder: immediate and short-term results. J Am Coll Cardiol 1998; 31(4): 878–82.

Meier B. Closure of patent foramen ovale: technique, pitfalls, complications, and follow up. Heart 2005; 91(4): 444–8. Review. No abstract available.

Mills NL, King TD. Late follow-up of nonoperative closure of secundum atrial septal defects using the King-Mills double-umbrella device. Am J Cardiol 2003; 92(3): 353–5.

Wahl A, Kunz M, Moschovitis A *et al.* Long-term results after fluoroscopy-guided closure of patent foramen ovale for secondary prevention of paradoxical embolism. Heart 2008; 94(3): 336–41. Epub 2007 July 16.

Index

Note: Page number in *italics* indicate pages with figures, page numbers in **bold** indicate pages with tables.